Music Heard So Deeply:
A Music Therapy Memoir

Betsey King, PhD, MT-BC

Published by BookLocker.com, Inc., Bradenton, Florida, U.S.A.

Printed on acid-free paper.

Prelude Music Therapy
2015

First Edition

for my parents

…or music heard so deeply
That it is not heard at all, but you are the music
While the music lasts.
-- T.S. Eliot, Four Quartets

TABLE OF CONTENTS

PRELUDE

Last year I celebrated my 30th anniversary as a board-certified music therapist. When I made the choice to pursue this vocation, in 1980, most people had never heard of the field. Many of the professors and coaches at the conservatory where I was studying violin performance thought I was insane – and a bit ungrateful – to consider a master's degree in such an unknown profession. Today, 35 years later, music therapy is a subject of feature reports in newspapers and on television, and books like Oliver Sacks' *Musicophilia* and Daniel Levitin's *This is Your Brain on Music* have tapped into the public's fascination with the way music affects the body, mind, and spirit.

Still, there remains a great deal of confusion about music therapy. Most people recognize the impact of music in their lives : from the lullabies that calm babies to the up-tempo beats that help make exercise easier. Many health care and education facilities bring music into their environments. Children memorize academic facts through songs and raps, hospital patients and families appreciate the music played at bedsides, and elderly residents in long-term care enjoy singing and dancing to their favorite tunes. Music is clearly beneficial. But music therapy is something else – something more.

Music therapy is the use of music by a certified professional to address specific, personal needs. It is based on assessment and evaluated through data. The music in music therapy is live, flexible, and responsive. Therapists and their clients build relationships through shared music. Music therapy is based on research but relies also on a therapist's intuition and creativity. It has roots in ancient practice while being supported by revolutionary brain-imaging research.

Music therapy as a profession was established here in the United States in 1950. There are rigorous standards for education and clinical training, a national certification program, and a growing number of state licenses. Despite this, the term "music therapy" is often applied by the news media to any use of music in healthcare or special education. It's frustrating. We are a relatively small profession without the resources for large marketing campaigns to share the research and experience we have. It is hard for people to understand the complexities and nuances of weaving music and therapy together.

Most of the published books about music therapy are academic or practical texts for music therapy professionals. This book is different. In one sense, I have written it for myself, as a record -- a scrapbook -- of the remarkable experiences I've been fortunate to have. Although my colleagues will recognize many of the feelings and events, it is no one's story but my own.

Mostly, though, I have written it to tell people about music therapy -- to share experiences and knowledge with people who are curious about how music affects us; those who know there is something about music that is more than what happens in a concert hall, arena, or playlist. If that is you, then I think you'll be fascinated with how music therapists work, be excited about what happens in a music therapy session, and be convinced that music therapy should be a part of any healthcare endeavor.

NOTES

This book is a series of clinical stories from my own experience as a board-certified music therapist (MT-BC), as well as some personal history and memories. Here and there I write about the theory or research that supports the work -- but this is not meant to be an academic text, so I have deliberately chosen to include it only where it explains how music therapists think or what motivated me to try something. I have chosen to tell the stories in a sequence that will explain aspects of music therapy, so the chapters are not in chronological order. If you want to keep track, it will be helpful to know that I was born near Chicago, studied violin in Cincinnati, studied music therapy in Dallas where I then practiced and taught for 20 years, did my doctoral work in Lawrence, Kansas, and then relocated to Rochester, New York for my current teaching position. The clinical stories which focus on the clients and the therapy process are, for the most part, separate from interludes which describe my own growth and experiences. At the end there are helpful links and reading suggestions if you want to know more.

Confidentiality is critical to any therapeutic profession, so I have taken care to protect identities by changing the names of my clients and altering details that don't have an impact on the truth of the story. I have not compressed any time in therapy: if I describe something as happening in a single session, that is how it happened. I have, in one case, placed sessions from different times into a single day for narrative purposes.

I've been fortunate to have worked in many different settings and circumstances. I practiced for many years in an acute rehabilitation hospital, with patients who had survived traumatic brain injuries, strokes, and other neuromuscular trauma -- and did regular sessions in the general hospital units while I was there. I spent four years as a full-time music therapist in a public school special education system and many other years doing contract work with people who have developmental disabilities. I often had small contracts for just a few hours with an agency or program, as when I worked at retreats for women with breast cancer. I substituted for other therapists occasionally and gained additional experience that way, and I sometimes introduced music therapy into a facility so that students where I was teaching could have experience with their clients; this is how I came to do music therapy work in settings like a pediatric emergency department and a county jail. Many music therapists work in a single setting for most of their career. That just isn't how my life progressed. As a college professor I am grateful for the breadth of experiences I have had so that I can share them with my students.

All music therapists complete certain steps for all their clients. (I will use the words "client" and "patient" at different points in this book; usually a "client" will be a person I see in a clinic or in the home, and a "patient" will be someone who I see in a medical or inpatient psychiatric setting. If I need one term for everyone, I will use "client.") We receive clients through referral and always complete an assessment to see if music therapy is likely to be effective. In some cases that assessment takes place over several sessions; in other cases, as when we might see a client only once, it is completed within the first few minutes of a session. Regardless, once the assessment is complete, we make a plan to accomplish something based on our observations, the available research, information from the health care team, and our intuition as therapists and musicians. We track progress, collect data, and document everything. We make adjustments within the sessions and between them. Finally, when goals have been met, or a client is discharged, or therapy is ending for any reason, we go through a process of closure with the client. I completed these steps for all the clients and patients described in this book, though I don't describe every step in every story. This also applies to other daily/hourly tasks like hand washing and disinfecting instruments.

There are some aspects of healthcare and therapy work that are perhaps difficult to understand. I have spent many years working with people who, through a traumatic accident or illness, have been irrevocably changed and impaired. The tragedy of "before" and "after" is profound and can be overwhelmingly sad. As a therapist, however, I always find myself relating solely to the person I am with at the time; I find my patients to be interesting people to get to know exactly as they are, even as we work to improve their lives. From that perspective, there can be humor without disrespect of the person, enjoyment without denial of the challenge.

Another aspect of the work that seems strange at first is that I rarely know what happens to my clients after I stop seeing them. When patients are discharged from the hospital, or special education students stop receiving music therapy, or I move away and leave a facility, I usually do not have the opportunity to keep in touch with them – nor would it be practical to do so. Over the past 30 years, I have worked with hundreds of clients and patients in three states and dozens of facilities. During therapy, I am fully engaged. Afterwards, I must move on so I can be present and focused on my next clients. For a therapist who works in the same agency or area for his or her whole career, this might be different. In my case, I can rarely tell anyone "how it all turned out in the end." The clinical stories in this book are like that. They tell you what happened in the sessions, but not what happened afterwards.

Finally, you will notice some aspects of the stories that will seem antiquated in current terms, particularly references to technology. I used cassette tapes for recordings for many years before CDs were developed. I wrote reports and created visual aids without a computer. The electronic piano keyboards I used for many years seemed revolutionary at the time; today they would be sold at a garage sale for $5. My current work involves a tablet, laptop, and mp3 players – and some music therapists work with even more sophisticated technology. But at the core of music therapy is live, acoustic music and the relationship we develop with our clients. Hopefully you will see that in these stories, no matter how old they are!

CHAPTER ONE

Sam

Alzheimer's disease and many forms of dementia are a tragedy for everyone involved. They rob people not just of their ability to remember and process their daily lives, they take their ability to communicate, plan, follow instructions, and control their emotions. They take away independence and put up barriers to the most important relationships. With an ever growing elderly population around the world, researchers and clinicians are fighting Alzheimer's and dementia with research on pharmaceuticals, genetics, care plans, and therapeutic interventions.

For people with dementia or Alzheimer's, music can sometimes seem like a miracle. Elders who can't recognize family members can recall and sing familiar songs, even play instruments. Anxiety can turn to joy in dancing. Drumming can stimulate interaction.

Recently, there has been a great deal of interest in the use of iPods with elders who have dementia or Alzheimer's disease. These seniors, listening to personalized playlists, often show increased energy, attention, and interaction with others. This is what I would call "therapeutic music" – it can be beneficial, but it's not music therapy. The music involvement is limited to listening and there isn't a music therapist there to take a person's responses and build them into something more. This session from my clinical practice shows what happens when that personal therapeutic relationship does occur, and the music can change and evolve.

February
Rochester, New York

I hurried up the stairs of the Music House, the former residence that became offices for music department faculty at Nazareth College. I unlocked the door of my office and exchanged the bag of books and notes I brought from class for my regular tote. Into the oversized purse I threw a small notebook of songs, my tablet and a miniature speaker. My guitar was already in my car. I was off to see my only private client at his home -- a session which was one of the highlights of my week.

Most of the therapy I have a chance to do as an associate professor occurs at our college's on-campus clinic, a training ground for our students. In 2012, however, I met a woman who was advocating for persons with Alzheimer's disease and she asked me to assess her husband, Sam, who had been diagnosed several years earlier. Once I had completed the assessment and it was clear he would benefit from music therapy, I agreed to stay on as his therapist. It wasn't that I had extra time to fill (any professor knows how ridiculous that is) but we were beginning to focus on Alzheimer's research at our college, and Sam's response to music was profound and joyful. It was also evident that Sam was responsive to my style of therapy.

Every music therapist has his or her own style. This is inevitable: we are musicians and we work in a profession for which relationship is a key component. If every MT-BC (board-certified music therapist) presented a song in exactly the same way, we would be no different than a recording. And while there are researched therapeutic techniques we learn and use, we relate to our clients as ourselves. Some music therapists are naturally quiet and gentle; they may lean towards work that benefits from those characteristics then make the extra effort to be more energetic when clients need that. Some music therapists find they do their best work within the structure of protocols: behavioral plans or medical procedures that need to remain consistently presented and require specific, often complex sets of cues.

My strengths as a therapist come from energy and humor. I can work in other styles, and do, but I work especially well with clients who respond to smiles and laughter and broad gestures. I have learned over the years how to present information slowly but enthusiastically and this works well with clients who have both cognitive challenges and the need to maintain focus and alertness. Sam was such a client and from our first assessment session, his wife, his aide and I all noticed that he was delighted to sing with a musician who had a bit of sass. He responded in kind, showing parts of his personality that had been missing in action, and I decided I should stay on as his therapist and fit his session into an already crazy schedule. It wasn't a sacrifice. I enjoyed each session as much as he did.

***

"Mr. G!" I exclaimed as did each time I entered the large living area where Sam sat in his favorite chair, "I've brought the music!" Sam put down the paper he had been holding (but was unable to read) and said "Ok." It was an automatic response; he wasn't able to anticipate my arrival or remember my name. I pulled up a chair in front of him and, as quickly as I could, got my guitar out of its case, speaking as few words as possible so that our first significant communication would be musical. I loved my old, worn guitar for one particular feature: it stayed in tune. This meant that I could almost always begin a session quickly, even if I had no time to set up.

Sam was sitting quietly, not completely sure what was about to happen. I strummed a single chord and, making sure Sam and I were looking at each other, began singing the Jones and Kahn song with which I almost always started.

"It had to be...."

"YOU!" shouted Sam, smiling and thrusting his pointed finger at me as he leaned forward. With the first chords and words, he sat up and in just that one moment, he was fully engaged.

It had to be you;
It had to be you!
I wandered around,
and finally found
the somebody who
could make me be true;
could make me feel blue,
and even be glad, just to be sad,
thinking of you...

I used a swing accompaniment style and kept the pace of the song moving forward, but used rubato (a slight rhythmic flexibility, often slowing for just a moment) and pauses so that Sam could fill in lyrics. I also used lots of gestures. It can take some trial and error to maintain the guitar accompaniment while taking one's hands away to indicate a lyric like "wandered around." I was relieved that at this point it came naturally, because I loved the way the gestures kept Sam alert. Sam imitated many of my movements automatically, but also remembered some of them from previous sessions and did them on his own, like pointing to his temple, then at me, for "thinking of you!"

Sam had a degenerative disease, but along with other clients I'd seen who have Alzheimer's or dementia, Sam was able to learn new things and remember them from session to session when they were structured with music.

Most of his recall was what could be called procedural memory, like memory for how to tie one's shoes, or write one's name -- something that once started can be finished automatically. Sam couldn't tie his shoes or sign his name anymore, but given the structure of rhythm and harmony, and a push from the melody, he would show me that he remembered a song, a gesture, or a short routine.

We started with *It Had to Be You* because it was our "contact song." Edith Boxill, who was a music therapist in New York City, wrote about this concept in a textbook on working with children with significant developmental disabilities. When a music therapist first starts to be musical with a client, she searches for that music -- the tempo, key, melody, rhythm, song -- that connects in such a way that she is not just playing *for* the client, but is playing *with* the client. Instead of one person initiating everything and waiting for a response, there is give and take: musical communication.

During my first assessment session with Sam, I played several songs for him, all my choices based on his wife's suggestions and on his age and background. He smiled and occasionally tapped his right hand on his leg during the first three, but the instant I started *It Had To Be You*, he sat up and exclaimed "You!" in a loud voice. More than that, the energy between us was, for the first time, an interchange --- energy was exchanged rather than given from me to him. This kind of connection doesn't have to be obvious or boisterous. I've worked with clients whose responses were imperceptible unless you were watching or listening for them: a movement of the eyes, an increase in the heartbeat, a tightening of a muscle. When I am in the attitude of making music *with* my client, I can begin to understand which responses are random and which are part of our communication.

With Sam, there was no need for interpretation, however. He let me know when he was engaged in the music. His face lit up, he leaned forward, he gestured or tapped his leg in rhythm. And once he was engaged in the music, he often became flirtatious. The deterioration in the frontal lobe of his brain (part of the course of Alzheimer's) meant that he didn't have the impulse control he used to -- so when we sang songs about love, Sam was happy to suggest that he and I might act out the song lyrics. He had lost much of his vocabulary, but he got his point across! I often had seen family members and caregivers try to correct this, but in our sessions I found that a combination of humor and redirecting Sam into the music -- getting him to sing a certain phrase, or emphasize the lyrics with a gesture, or play an instrument -- was more effective than trying to get him to stop. The right music is a powerful magnet.

With our first song wrapping up, I grabbed the bongo drums I had with me. I was working with Sam on initiating movement and then controlling it; each skill involving at least two distinct networks in the brain. The song we used for this was *Red Red Robin*. Each line of lyrics emphasized the first three strong beats of the four-beat measures.

When the <u>red</u> <u>red</u> <u>rob</u>in comes
<u>bob</u>-<u>bob</u>-<u>bob</u>bin'
a<u>long</u> * *,
a<u>long</u> * *

There'll be <u>no</u> <u>more</u> <u>sob</u>bin'
When <u>he</u> <u>starts</u> <u>throb</u>bin' his
<u>old</u> * * sweet
<u>song</u>...

When I first assessed Sam on playing a beat, he showed me immediately that he had a strong sense of a song's rhythm; in fact, he usually attempted to beat most of the notes in the melody and showed some control (he didn't just beat randomly). I could tell that an impulse to reproduce the melody through beating the drum was automatic for him. That was great -- a wonderful indication of something preserved in Sam. I wanted to work for something more, though: more deliberate playing, more awareness of cooperating with another person. I wanted to preserve his ability to control his actions and interactions as long as possible.

So, using one of the pair of bongos for myself, I started singing, and beat the first three beats forcefully ("Red! Red! Rob!in) -- then pushed the other side of the bongos towards Sam. During the previous two weeks, Sam had needed a visual cue from me, but this week he reached out immediately and hit the drum for three strong beats of his own (Bob! Bob! Bob!ing). Back to me for three, over to Sam, who again played his three. Whoo Hoo! This was an improvement and I took note of it for the data I would record later. The song then moved into a section that was a chance for us to sing in call-and-response with repeated lyrics:

Wake up! Wake up! (you sleepyhead!)
Get up! Get up! (Get out of bed!)
Cheer up! Cheer up! (The sun is red)
Live! Love! Laugh and be happy...

Sam always repeated "Wake up!" easily, but like many people with mid- and later-stage Alzheimer's or dementia, he could get stuck on a word or phrase, and he might repeat "Wake up" instead of moving on to the other lyrics. However, I'd found that if I added some complexity to the harmony at the end of the first phrase, or add some bass notes, Sam was more likely to listen to me sing "Get up!" and correctly repeat it. This fit with research that shows more complex harmony increasing alertness and strong bass rhythms increasing responsiveness. Of course, nothing about the way Sam and I sang this song seemed like a controlled experiment. We sang and shouted at each other, laughing. "Cheer up!" "Cheer up!"

There were subtle, quieter moments that were worth noting, too. As we sang our third song of the session, Sam's attention drifted in the middle of our second run-through. I had been playing the relatively steady strummed accompaniment in 4/4 time, but when I saw his eyes wander and his mouth slacken a bit, I ended the next phrase with a strong downbeat followed by three beats of silence under the lyrics. I picked up the pattern again right away, but that simple short interruption captured his attention and by the next line of lyrics, we were in the music together again. For me, that moment was like improvising in jazz or making subtle changes in chamber music: my fellow musician had done something different and I responded musically.

We had completed three fairly lively songs, so I chose a quieter one. One of our goals was for Sam to actively focus for as much of a 40 minute session as possible. I didn't want him to wear himself out or become overstimulated. I began the gentle accompaniment for *What a Wonderful World*, incorporating gestures for major lyrics. As he had in previous weeks, Sam listened more than sang, but he followed the gestures attentively, occasionally imitating them.

I see trees of green
Red roses, too
I see them bloom
for me and you
and I think to myself:
What a Wonderful World...

As I completed the title line and continued the accompaniment, Sam leaned forward and said "But do you think it is?"

This was startling. Sam's Alzheimer's disease had led to aphasia -- a language disorder -- so Sam didn't initiate conversation, and he had a great deal of difficulty understanding conversations around him. He did not make independent, on-topic contributions like this. The familiarity of the music and his immersion in it clearly had stimulated him. I hesitated for a moment in surprise, with my inner voice yelling, "Don't just sit there, say something!"

"Well," I said, "Most days have disappointments, but overall I do think it's a wonderful world."

Sam nodded. "Exactly," he said, gesturing towards the guitar.

I wanted to see if the conversation could continue. "Do you think it is a wonderful world?" I asked.

He gestured at the guitar. "You ...said it," he responded, haltingly. The moment was over. I took up the song again and Sam resumed his listening and gestures. I realized that part of my brain was already adding this surprise to the progress note I would be writing and I had to inwardly poke myself to put my full attention on Sam in the present moment.

Our penultimate song was one that I'd chosen and designed to focus on memory and picture recognition. Both of these were skills that were waning for Sam, and I wanted to stimulate those neural networks to maintain as much of Sam's ability as possible. A song from his favorite genre worked well for this: *They Can't Take That Away from Me*.

I had a recording of Ella Fitzgerald and Louis Armstrong on my tablet as well as a gallery of pictures for many of the major words in the lyrics. I plugged my portable speaker into the tablet and cued up the song, quickly following that by pulling up the gallery and getting ready to show Sam the first picture. As usual, I scrolled through the pictures during the first run-through of the song, just letting Sam see and hear the lyrics. Music doesn't work as a context for skill work if your client doesn't experience the whole song. You can't fill in the blanks if you don't know the words! Some clients will remember a whole song on their own and you can break it apart for a task right away, but a person with Alzheimer's or dementia needs to get re-acquainted with the music each session.

The introduction played and Ella began singing.

The way you wear your hat
The way you sip your tea
The memory of all that
No, no! They can't take that away from me!
The way your smile just beams

The way you sing off-key
The way you haunt my dreams
No, no! They can't take that away from me!

During this run-through, I made some gestures and sang along. Sam's favorite thing to do each week was to respond to the little finger wag gesture I made for "No, no" and give me a real talking-to: "No, no, no, no, no, no, NO!" he sang, leaning forward and waving a finger in front of my face, grinning the whole time. This obliterated the recording and we always missed the beginning of the next phrase, but his joy -- and the evidence of his alertness -- was worth it.

Once we heard the recording and saw the pictures, I sang the song live, pausing on each key word. Sam had "hat" down pat, was improving on "tea" (it was sometimes "cup" and sometimes "coffee"), and could get "smile" and "dreams" if he heard me start to sound out the words. Best of all, the energy he got from his "no no no!" carried over and he sang almost all the words to the title line. He had trouble with "c" in "can't" (sounds produced from the back of the mouth/throat are more difficult) but once I sang "They can't..." he completed it with "take...that...away....from....me." I slowed the tempo down for this phrase and made sure my mouth didn't involuntarily form the syllables, and I could see him working on each word. This kind of deliberation was exactly what we wanted; it indicated that he was not just repeating something automatically (one neural network), but was recalling each word and putting them in order (a different network). When he succeeded this time, I couldn't keep myself from cheering. "Whoo hoo! Sam! That was great!" Sam gave me a smile that seemed to say, "What a goofball. What is all the fuss about?"

Sam and I finished every session with a song suggested by his wife -- one I would not have thought to introduce otherwise: *Don't Fence Me In*. Sam came to this country from Eastern Europe after surviving in a work camp during the Holocaust, and he had loved American cowboys like Roy Rogers. As usual, I sang most of the song, using a Texas twang, and left the title line for Sam. He sang it with gusto.

Give me land, lots of land,
under starry skies above,
Don't Fence Me In!
Let me ride through the wide open
country that I love,
Don't Fence Me In!

Sam patted his leg in rhythm and got ready for the big finish.

Let me be by myself in the evening breeze
Listen to the murmur of the cottonwood trees
Send me off forever but I ask you please:

(and now Sam sang each word higher than the previous one)

Don't FENCE ME IN!!

And yes, I got the irony, even if Sam didn't. Perhaps that's why this was one of the best parts of my week. I had experienced dementia in my own family; I knew that the day-to-day care is almost always a terrible strain, a reminder of loss, and a type of prison. But here I got to smile and laugh and sing with this lovely man and I knew it gave his wife some joy to hear this part of him express itself. I knew that his participation in music likely was prolonging his ability to communicate. And I knew how lucky I was to be present for moments like the ones Sam experienced in music therapy.

CHAPTER TWO

The Emergency Department

Many hospitals today are recognizing that music can be a positive addition to a healthcare environment. Some have musicians come and play for their patients and families. Most now have some way for patients to play recorded music in their hospital rooms. This is a wonderful acknowledgment of the important part music plays in our lives. Still, outside of pediatrics (where music therapists are more common), music in healthcare is still primarily a volunteer effort or one that only offers music "at bedside" -- calming music played by a performer. For some patients, this is all that is needed. But if the hospital doesn't have a music therapist, patients in need don't have access to someone trained to develop treatment plans for specific symptoms and track responses.

There are myriad ways in which music therapy can be effective in a medical setting. Research supports the use of music in units like the neonatal ICU, pediatrics, rehabilitation, cardiac care, oncology, and surgery, but each medical system must find a way to pay for it -- and most don't. Even in the areas where research has demonstrated that music therapy reduces the need for medication, decreases the length of hospital stays, or improves outcomes, insurance coverage is rare. Yet a single music therapist (with a single salary) can have an impact on multiple units of a hospital, benefiting both patients and staff. This is the story of just a single afternoon spent in the pediatric emergency department of a metropolitan hospital. Reading about this and the other medical cases in this book, imagine the impact multiplied into a full week, or a month, or a year throughout an entire medical center.

November
Rochester, New York

The pediatric emergency department was obviously busy when my student and I arrived on Wednesday afternoon. We were there to fill in for the hospital's music therapist who was out with a hand injury. I had just moved to the area become an assistant professor in the local college degree program. This was both a good way to get involved in the community and an excellent place for one of our students to do some clinical training. After we were buzzed into the treatment area, with our guitars in soft cases over our shoulders and bags of instruments in our hands, we had to thread our way past two empty stretchers and one doctor-parent conference on our way to the nurses' station. The charge nurse looked over the list of names in front of her and pointed us to Room 4 down the hall. "They've been here for an hour already," she said, "and I'll bet they would like the entertainment."

Having music therapy in the pediatric "E.D." was new for the hospital; the regular music therapist had only made one visit before her injury. That meant that few of the staff knew anything about it, and might have thought we were supposed to be there as entertainment. Having had varied experiences with doctors and nurses over the years, I wasn't sure whether we would be welcomed, seen as a curiosity, or viewed as a nuisance. My student Christine, meanwhile, was nervous about her first clinical training experience in a medical facility. Lots of uncertainty followed us into the treatment room.

Our first patient was a young boy, about 8 years old. He and his mother were waiting for a doctor to check back in; the boy had received stitches and a shot earlier and he needed to be checked before they could leave. I entered the room alone because I didn't want a child to be overwhelmed by adults. Christine was ready to wait just outside the door until I gave her a signal. I introduced myself.

"Hi. My name is Betsey. I'm a music therapist. We bring music to the rooms here, to help with the waiting and maybe help you relax. Could we play a little bit for you?"

It wasn't unusual to provide a simplified explanation of our role to start, especially for children. Once I finished my assessment -- which in single visits like this I would do in the first few minutes -- I could provide a more specific goal for the music therapy session.

The boy's name was Chad. His mother invited us in, but Chad didn't acknowledge us. He was looking at a book filled with pictures of cars, trucks and motorcycles. He was fidgety and probably anxious to go home, but he was uninterested in the idea of listening to or playing music. His mother, who perhaps wondered if they were required to participate, tried encouraging him to talk to me, but I reassured her that it was perfectly okay for him to turn me down. I chatted with her for a few minutes so Chad could see the instruments and get used to me, just in case he only needed some time to decide. He didn't show any interest. Music therapy isn't always needed.

From across the hall came the wailing of a very young patient and, as it continued, the frustrated and increasingly loud voice of a young woman. It seemed that she was losing her ability to stay calm. I said goodbye to Chad and his mother and slipped across the hall.

"Hi," I said, making eye contact with the girl who turned out to be the little patient's mother. She had her son facing her on her lap and he was struggling and crying, a breathing mask over his mouth and nose. She looked ready to shake him in frustration. "I'm a music therapist here at the hospital. Maybe I can help calm him down with some music. Would you like for me to try?"

She looked visibly relieved and nodded. I told Christine to go back to the nurses' station and tell them where we would be.

The little guy, Jordan, was 2 years old and receiving treatment for an asthma attack. He was crying inconsolably, his chubby little arms flying up and down. I called Christine in and told her to grab a paddle drum from my bag and an adapted mallet. A paddle drum looks like its name: a large round drum head with a handle. It has a nice resonance and the handle gives me a lot of flexibility in how I present the drum to patients. My mallet has a handle padded with plumber's insulation so it doesn't require as much of a tight grasp.

I was able to quickly open Jordan's flailing right hand and place the mallet's padded handle inside; he grabbed it automatically as his hand tensed up again, and now the mallet was going up and down in a regular rhythm, synchronized with his gulps of breath between cries. When Christine maneuvered the paddle drum to the right place, we heard a big beat every time his hand flew down. I started half-singing, half-chanting Jordan's name to the beat of his "drumming" and added lyrics about what we were doing.

Jordan, Jordan,
playing on the drum
Mom is holding him
and he's beating on the drum...

Once I'd established a basic eight-bar song in 4/4 time, I repeated it, keeping to Jordan's tempo. When I started the song for the third time, I began to slow the pace of the song almost imperceptibly every measure. Very gradually, I decreased the tempo and Jordan's beat slowed with me. Within a couple of minutes, his cries had gaps between them and the rhythm of both the cries and his drumbeat had slowed along with mine. Slower, quieter, slower....suddenly his eyes opened and he saw me and suddenly we were back at full volume, full speed crying, and flailing.

Ok. We started again; Jordan hadn't let go of the mallet, so Christine readjusted the drum position and I began singing "his" song again, eventually starting the gradual decrease in tempo. Again, Jordan slowed with me. This time, after a couple of minutes, we got all the way to quiet, Christine removing the drum from beneath his still hand and Jordan's mom stroking his back and talking softly to him.

Peace.

We all sat quietly for a minute or two, and then I began to strum the guitar as Jordan's mom and I talked. I learned that Jordan liked the songs in the children's shows he watched on tv, but that he also liked the soul and blues music his mom listened to. As we talked, Jordan watched us and when his mom took off the breathing mask, he began to babble along with our conversation. When I started a blues progression on the guitar, he smiled and began to move -- though much more like a dance than the flailing of earlier. I changed the rhythmic pattern I was using so there was a pause every measure. (If you say the phrase "beneath the bed" you'll hear the rhythm I was playing. Think "one, two" after the phrase and you'll hear the two-beat pause.) Each time, I played the pattern and then said "Hi!" to Jordan in the pause. He watched me intently.

When I had repeated the pattern 4 times, I started again, but left the space after without saying anything. In the pause I leaned towards him with an expectant look. He smiled. I leaned back, played the pattern again and leaned forward....

"AH!" he said.

"Bah DAH bah DAH," I played.

"AH!" he said, smiling.

And off we went, at a relaxed pace so as not to overstimulate our little patient. Christine picked up the drum and provided some gentle backup -- and then, suddenly, there was Jordan's mom with a beautiful voice, singing in response to her son.

"AH!" he exclaimed.
"Sweet boy!" she sang
"AH!"
"sweet sweet boy"
"AH"
"I hear you"
"AH"
"sweet, sweet boy"

The treatment room was alive with music.

We played and sang for several minutes, then had to stop because a nurse and doctor arrived and indicated it was time for Christine and me to move on. But thinking back to why we came into the room in the first place, I made sure to talk with Jordan's mom for a moment about what we did and how she might adapt it at home. I told her, truthfully, that her singing was wonderful and that it might be something that could help Jordan calm down when he got upset. I didn't really think that we could change how they coped with stress in one short visit, but wanted to at least try to give her some ideas.

Christine and I headed back to the nurses' station where we were greeted with smiles. Several of the medical staff commented on what fun it was to hear the music down the hall and what a relief to hear the crying stop. We got an immediate request to go to a treatment room right across from the station. "That girl is having an asthma treatment and her mom is in with her. She got really upset earlier, so maybe the music would help her keep calm."

Already we were getting a more goal-directed referral!

Our new patient was 11 years old; she had long blond hair and was wearing a soccer outfit. She was lying in the bed and still suffering the after-effects of a severe asthma attack. She had a clear mask over her nose and mouth which was delivering medication, but we could see her chest rising and falling too quickly, her face showing her anxiety. Her mother sat in a chair on the other side of the bed, holding her daughter's right hand. I approached the bed and introduced myself and Christine to both our patient and her mother.

The mother was enthusiastic, the girl -- Marilinda -- hesitant but willing. I pulled my guitar out of the case and begin to improvise a song based on her name, using a pop ballad style. As with Jordan, I didn't worry about rhyming or matching the lyrics perfectly to the rhythm; I just tried to accurately reflect what our patient was thinking and feeling. The first lyrics came out this way:

Marilinda, Marilinda
We're singing your name
Marilinda, Marilinda,
The music is for you.

I continued the song, now changing the lyrics based on ideas from Marilinda and sometimes vocalizing the melody without words. As I did so, I asked Christine to get out some of the instruments we'd brought with us. Soon Marilinda was shaking a small maraca, her mother was tapping a tambourine, and Christine was providing a gentle beat with a drum. I maintained a tempo just a bit slower than Marilinda's breathing and watched as her respirations gradually slowed towards the tempo of the music. As we sang and played, I periodically pointed out our strategies to Marilinda's mother, showing her how

Marilinda's breathing was entraining to the music and how her expressions of anxiety were lessening.

The first twenty minutes of our time together passed with more singing, some talking about Marilinda's favorite music and activities, and trying out some of the other instruments we had, including a small glockenspiel with a rich, resonant sound. The nurse came in and out, checking on the level of medication remaining and taking readings. The music was distracting Marilinda, and relaxing her, but we were also establishing a relationship and a measure of trust.

This trust became important when the doctor arrived and told Marilinda that she needed to have an IV started. It became evident that Marilinda had been through this before; knowing that an IV meant the insertion of a needle into her arm, she started crying immediately, becoming agitated. This, of course, increased the speed of her breathing as she became more and more upset. As her mother comforted her, I began to play quietly on the guitar and soon, with doctor out of the room and the procedure apparently not imminent, Marilinda calmed down.

I knew it was important not to downplay her fears. She still needed to be able to express herself and we had established that the music was hers, reflecting her perspective. I kept the music quiet and began to sing the phrase she had been crying to the doctor: "I don't want it!" Then I added a line and after singing it twice asked if we could keep it in the song. She agreed, and sang with me, still with some tears in her eyes.

I don't want it
I don't want it
But my lungs say thank you
My lungs say thank you

We repeated this two times and then I moved into playing and singing *What a Wonderful World*, as I encouraged her to relax. Christine harmonized with me and the room became quiet apart from the music and the hissing sound of the medication flowing to Marilinda through her mask.

Ten minutes later, the nurse and two aides arrived, ready to insert the IV and obviously ready for a struggle on the part of their patient. And indeed, when she saw them, Marilinda began to cry and twist away from her mother, becoming more hysterical by the second. I knew the research showing music therapy is effective as a procedural support in medical settings, and I hoped that the relationship I had built with my patient would be helpful now. As the nurse and aides moved to Marilinda's right side to insert the IV, her mother moved to Marilinda's left and stroked her hair. Meanwhile, I encouraged Marilinda to keep her eyes on her mother and me, and I began to sing the song we'd practiced.

I don't want it;
I don't want it
But my lungs say thank you
My lungs say thank you.

Marilinda did not visibly calm down. The aides had to hold her arms, and she continued to cry and pull away. My student, Christine, shrank back at the hysteria in the girl's voice. It was easy to assume that the music was having no effect.

But I remembered Dave, a patient I'd worked with during my time at a rehabilitation hospital. Dave had been severely injured in a helicopter crash and his physical therapy, stretching muscles that had contracted after the accident, had been excruciating for him. His cries and moans filled the physical therapy gym during his half-hour sessions. His physical therapist began to feel the physical and emotional strain of their work, too. She and Dave decided to see if music could help him through the stretching. So, for two weeks, I attended the physical therapy sessions at which he had to kneel, raise up through his thighs and place his forearms on top of a large bolster, straightening from his neck to his knees. I knelt opposite him, put my forearms on the bolster and we looked at each other as we sang his favorite 60's folk songs. Often he was singing through gritted teeth, sometimes he was shouting the lyrics, and most of the time he was sweating up a storm. Still, he asked me to come back time after time and when he was discharged to outpatient care, he told me, "Thank God for the music. I don't know what I would have done without it."

So I knew that it was possible that the music was helping Marilinda, and I kept singing, and finally the IV was in. She gradually stopped crying, but after the nurses and aides left she began to complain that the needle site was painful. "It's hurting me! It hurts!" she sobbed. I gave her the mallet for the glockenspiel she had been playing earlier, and told her, "Every time it hurts you, hit this as hard as you can." Her first two smacks at the instrument were ferocious, but they became less so as she kept playing. Then, as I started playing a more upbeat accompaniment on my guitar and encouraged her to write some lyrics about how brave she had been, and how much better she was going to feel, she stopped playing and talking about the pain altogether.

Soon afterwards, the doctor made the decision to transfer her to the city's primary children's hospital, and I had Marilinda help me write lyrics about what this would be like. We wrote a verse about the stretcher (and how she didn't want the straps too tight), and about the attendants who would take her (and how we hoped they'd be cute guys!), and then, as we talked about the ambulance, Marilinda herself brought back a thread from the very first song about her name, and sang:

Marilinda, Marilinda,
Going in an ambulance
Taking music with me

The music is for me.

I felt a rush of happiness. How wonderful to hear her taking what we'd offered and making it her own.

As Marilinda was being moved to the gurney and handling it well, her mother approached us. "Thank you," she said. "That helped so much."

"I hope so," I said, "but I know the IV procedure was tough on her."

The nurse interrupted. "No, you don't understand," she told us. "It went so much smoother today. That was the easiest it's ever been." Marilinda's mother nodded in agreement. "I wish there could be music here every time we have an IV put in."

"Me, too!" said the nurse.

After we signed out of the emergency department, my student and I debriefed. The afternoon had provided a wealth of information for Christine. She'd seen that music therapy wasn't always necessary, she'd observed the benefits of a toddler's involuntary and alert responses to rhythm, and she had experienced the power of music to build trust and safety for a scared pre-teen. We both felt that the medical staff had begun to understand the difference between music as entertainment and music as therapy.

INTERLUDE

What is Music Therapy?

A graduate professor once told me that the question isn't "What is music therapy?" but rather, "Who is music therapy?" He had a point. Music therapy, like other therapeutic professions, has theories and principles, procedures and protocols. Becoming a music therapist requires university study, clinical training, and certification. Within the profession are distinct schools of thought and a variety of post-graduate training institutes.

But it's easier, and clearer, to define the field by talking about music therapists.

Music therapists are, first and last, musicians -- but while they may play or sing as performers in part of their lives, they do not perform as a part of therapy. Instead, they share music, involving their clients in playing and singing, listening and moving, to help them reach specific goals. Music therapists have a heightened sense of music as communication because they don't simply play or sing *to* someone; they are successful only when that person becomes active in the musical experience, often revealing an ability or emotion that might not be seen otherwise.

Music therapists use live music. They play the piano, or guitar, or percussion, and they are ready, moment to moment, to change the tempo or key or other aspect of the music to match a person's mood or energy level. They prepare some music in advance, choosing or composing it for an individual need, and improvise other music on the spot, reflecting and affirming the person before them. They know that everyone responds to music differently, and that one size does not fit all. Because of this, they do not promote their music to the public with grandiose promises of healing or educational benefits. In fact, most music therapists don't think beyond the unique needs of the people in the hospital, school, nursing home, veterans' center, hospice, or practice where they work. They share their ideas and strategies through books and journals and conferences.

Music therapists are specifically educated and certified, and their training is rigorous. (All qualified music therapists in the U.S. are designated "MT-BC" – Music Therapist, Board Certified.") For most of them, their preparation begins years before college, as they learn to play an instrument or use their voice, both as soloists and in ensembles. Then they must attend an approved college or university program which will include music, academic, and clinical education. This will culminate in an internship which often lasts half a year or more, and if they graduate successfully, they will take a national certification exam and maintain their certification with continuing education. Many will continue onto advanced degrees, some to additional certification in specialized areas of practice.

Some music therapists are researchers, carefully examining the effects of music and music therapy interventions in experimental and experiential settings. Most music therapists are clinicians with a caseload of individual and group sessions, but even then they work with a research mindset, attending to each detail of their sessions and making changes based on what they observe. They document their work in order to track its effectiveness and are challenged each day to balance paperwork, session planning, and music practice.

Music therapists are collaborative. Working with educators, for example, they help children with autism deal with sensory and social challenges. Working with physical therapists, they help people with Parkinson's disease move with more fluidity and safety. Working with doctors and nurses, they help patients with cancer cope with the symptoms and emotional toll of the disease and its treatments. Many work in private practice, but always with an awareness of all of the influences in a patient's or client's life.

Music therapists seek to help others. Most start with vague personal convictions about music's ability to "help people" which are tempered and strengthened and changed by their training and education. Music therapists study the physical and psychological factors that keep people from reaching their full potential, but they accept each person without judgment. They can take whatever a person can do, however small, and include it a part of a satisfying musical whole.

Music therapists use the elements of music, such as melody, harmony, rhythm, timbre -- and activities of music like singing, playing instruments, creating, moving, and listening -- to effect change for their clients. When the triangle of therapist, client, and music comes together in music therapy, it can spark physiological changes, improve cognitive functioning, spur increases in communication, support improved social skills, and touch emotional and spiritual depths. This is not done surreptitiously, as when a grocery store plays music in the hope that you will linger, but rather in an open plan of therapy with specific goals and objectives. Music therapists watch for the outward signs of progress while knowing that music can find and heal inner wounds and private pain.

Music therapists are artists and scientists, but they must be educators, too, because many people still do not know what music therapy is. Advocacy is still a part of almost every music therapist's job. This book is part of that.

CHAPTER THREE

The Rehab Hospital

The use of music therapy in physical medicine rehabilitation has changed since I was the music therapist at an acute rehabilitation hospital. Before managed care -- which includes the system in which a diagnosis is tied to a total amount of money that can be spent on care and treatment -- each patient's treatment program was determined individually. If an assessment showed that music therapy would be effective for a patient's goals, it was ordered by the physician, even if the patient was already receiving several other types of therapy. Patient stays were longer, too, and determined primarily by the treatment team. Today, however, rehabilitation funds are limited and approved programs often only include three primary therapies: physical, occupational, and speech/language.

For me, the best part of working in rehab was the teamwork. Research supports the effectiveness of interprofessional work, and rehabilitation medicine is often driven by a team rather than a single doctor. This provides a learning experience for each member of the team. Reading about splints or standing frames or communication devices is one thing: working with the therapists and patients who are using them is another, and rehabilitation team members are often working close to one another, in adjoining treatment areas. When a music therapist is part of the team, the other therapists and medical staff have the chance to see how music therapy can provide a unique motivation and a significant assist in neurological recovery for some patients.

Another aspect of rehabilitation work I enjoyed was the variety. Rehab patients are people of all ages and backgrounds, cultures and interests, and each injury results in specific and distinct challenges. Once again, the importance of providing music therapy rather than generic music recreation is evident; no one type of music or one kind of musical interaction can be effective in improving patients' recoveries. This chapter has three stories describing three different uses of music for three completely different goals.

June
Dallas, Texas

On Tuesday, one of the aides at the rehabilitation hospital brought Andy to his fourth, and last, music therapy session. I had been asked by the rehab team to see if music therapy would help Andy become more alert and more responsive. In our first three sessions, Andy had shown little to no interest in, or reaction to, music and I didn't expect to see any difference on this last day of the assessment period. Music therapy is not for everyone.

But sometimes therapists need to try something completely different.

Andy had survived a traumatic brain injury, received in a car crash. He was 52 years old, a husband, and father to two grown children. His family had told the team that Andy led a conservative life, working hard, maintaining personal discipline and setting boundaries for his children. When asked about music, his son told me that the only music they were allowed to play in their home was classical or old-fashioned country-western.

Andy's brain injury was primarily located in the frontal lobe of his brain, and as can often be the case, the result was that he had significant problems with initiation and attention. He did not demonstrate any significant response to his environment or the people around him. His head slumped forward most of the time. The one impulse he had shown was to try and get out of his wheelchair. This was a problem, because he did not have control over his legs, and if he attempted to stand, he fell forward onto the floor. As a result, the staff had put Andy in a kind of smock: an open-back garment with sleeves. The smock had long cloth straps that could be tied to the wheelchair. These cloth ties were threaded around the back of the wheelchair to the front again and tied in a bow at the front of the smock at waist level.

The smock was a faded blue and red plaid. It was not a distinguished look. I had seen Andy looking down at the main knot tied in front of him and once or twice had seen him poke at it with his left hand. It was easy to imagine that he did not like wearing it or being seen in it, but there was no way for Andy to communicate that if it were true. His ability to speak had been severely impaired and he had not been able to use any communication tools like keyboards for typing words, or pictures to point at.

Andy's brain injury had also affected his arms and hands. He was naturally right handed, but his right arm was drawn up against his body and his right hand was curled up even more (This "decorticate posturing" is a sign of severe brain damage). He rarely moved either voluntarily. His left arm was stiff but he could extend it, and his left hand could open -- but I hadn't seen him do either in response to musical interventions.

So there we were, on this last day of music therapy, in the little treatment room I had off of the larger therapeutic recreation area in the basement of the rehab hospital. (Music therapy works best in its own room because the MT-BC needs to contrast music and silence.) I already knew that Andy did not respond to my singing, either familiar songs or songs I improvised about him and his family. I knew that he would not grasp a mallet or hold an instrument so I could play and let him feel the vibrations. He had not reached out towards anything in the room: my guitar, the large drum, the keyboard on its stand to his left. I had tried playing recordings of his favorite songs and singing them live, but couldn't see any change -- not in his breathing or heartbeat, not in his posture or expression.

On this last day, wanting so badly to give Andy a chance to communicate, I decided to try something radical. He hadn't responded to any of the music that was supposedly his preference, so I decided to think about the elements of music and how they can affect people. I knew a colleague of mine in Wisconsin had had success using deep bass notes to increase the attention of her adult clients with severe disabilities. I also knew that there was emerging research showing that strong rhythmic stimulation could prompt movement. With this in mind, I pulled Prince's "Purple Rain" tape off my shelf and cued up *Let's Go Crazy.*

I wanted to play it loudly and even with the door between us and the larger therapy area, I knew the music would distract patients outside, so I used an adapter that let Andy and me each wear headphones to listen. The track started with a voice, amplified with reverb. I watched Andy closely but there was no visible response. Thirty-five seconds in, a strong, pulsating beat started in under the voice. Almost immediately, Andy lifted his head and looked around. At 53 seconds the other instruments, including an electric guitar, came in and the track drove forward, aggressive and loud. I kept one hand on the volume knob, ready to turn it down if necessary. Compared to the music we had been listening to, this was cacophony. I watched Andy for any signs of distress at this onslaught, but instead what I saw was him nodding his head, eyes open, and a small smile from the left side of his lips. As the track continued, his posture improved and there was a slight movement of his torso side to side as his head continued to nod.

I had reasons for trying this, but I was still surprised. I mentally searched options for what could happen next to maintain Andy's focus. As the song moved forward, I pulled the electronic piano towards his wheelchair and removed his lap tray so the keyboard could be as close to him as possible. I knew that some really high and dissonant guitar riffs would occur near the end of the track, so I faded the song before that happened and simultaneously turned up the volume on the keyboard which I had set to play a rhythm like the one in the song. I held my breath, hoping that Andy would continue to be engaged.

Andy leaned forward, looking directly at the piano as the beat pushed on. He extended his left arm towards the keyboard and by leaning forward a bit more, he was able to put his left fist on the keys. A tight cluster of notes sounded, accompanied by the pulsating rhythm -- and because the keyboard was electronic, the sound continued without fading out. Waaaaaaaaaaaaaaaaaaaaa!

Andy lifted his fist and moved it to the left, pushed down, and sounded a lower group of notes. The volume was loud and all the notes so close together sounded quite dissonant, so I quickly plugged the headphones into the piano. Now only Andy and I were listening. Andy lifted his hand up again and twisted his wrist so that his thumb could play individual notes. Up and down, he moved around the lower half of the keyboard experimenting with notes. Then, quite deliberately, he moved back to playing clusters of notes. It was now clear that he could play single notes and remove his hand anytime but that he was choosing to play these "chord clusters" and keep the sound going.

Now something else was happening. Andy twisted his body, leaned forward, and stretched out his right arm towards the keyboard. He was having to work against greater tension in this arm; the right did not extend away from his body as far as the left, so he compensated by leaning forward until his right fist was able to drop onto the keys. He played a cluster of notes as before, slightly higher this time because he was reaching to the right side of the keyboard. And now, as the notes sounded, he began to reach his left arm back and down, towards his left foot. What was he doing?

As his left arm reached back, his body moved back with it and inevitably his right fist slid off the keyboard. The sounds stopped -- and so did Andy. He sat up, leaned forward, and once again got his right fist onto the keys. The cluster of notes started again and he again began trying to reach down and back with his left hand. Each time he tried this, he got a bit farther down, but at some point, the right hand always slid off the keyboard. Each time, he reset himself. I was befuddled as to what he was doing, but he was doing it with such intent that I didn't want to interrupt. None of us on Andy's team had seen this kind of focus.

Finally, on his fifth try, he achieved his goal -- and pulled his left shoe off of his foot. I had a brief moment to wonder what on earth was going on before he sat up again and with great effort, placed his shoe on the keys of the electronic keyboard. The shoe was heavy enough to depress the keys, so now the shoe was playing a cluster chord. And what did Andy do? He immediately moved both hands to the bow tied at the front of his smock and began working to untie it!

Wow. Nothing in Andy's prior behavior or responses had indicated that he would be able work on solving a problem like this. He had obviously responded to the strong rhythm and drive of *Let's Go Crazy* with more alertness. But why the cluster chords? To almost anyone's ears, in any culture, the simultaneous and sustained playing of several notes right next to each other is dissonant and often unpleasant. Yet Andy had not only deliberately played them but figured out a way to make sure a cluster chord continued to sound while he attempted to untie his smock. All I could guess was that for Andy, the injury to his brain and the resulting reduction in effective neural networks for attention and alertness meant that he required more intense auditory stimulation. "Pleasant" wasn't enough to cause his brain to respond.

Andy and I didn't get a chance to explore this further. An infection that had been responding to treatment flared up again and by the time he recovered, Andy's family (and probably their insurance agency) had made the decision to move him to a long-term facility where there was no music therapist. We would never have another music therapy session, but Andy had left me the gift of questions and ideas that I would continue to explore for years to come, including in my doctoral dissertation almost 10 years later.

***

It was not unusual, in acute rehabilitation, to have a patient who expressed suicidal thoughts or at least ambivalence about having survived a traumatic injury or illness. Facing a future with so many challenges and deficits was devastating. Trying to process this when one's cognitive abilities were damaged only added to the trauma. Those of us who were part of the healthcare system also knew that much more money was spent on sophisticated trauma responses than was available to care for our patients afterwards and for the rest of their lives. There wasn't adequate support for our patients' long-term physical recovery and management, much less their emotional healing.

"Y Me? Y didn't I die? Y didn't I stay in heaven?" one of my patients typed on her communication device (she was unable to speak after a traumatic brain injury). Aubrey had started the session expressing a specific desire to commit suicide, while despairing that her physical limitations would prevent her from doing it. In that session and others, we worked through several stages of her emotional response through talking, discussing song lyrics, and composing both instrumental music and songs. Music, in all its forms, can provide a place of safety as well as provocation. Lyrics from a popular song, for example, can allow people to explore scary topics by talking first about the person in the song rather than themselves. Other lyrics, or the emotions conveyed in the music, can provoke a deeper conversation.

Aubrey also benefitted from creating instrumental music: a score for the various parts of her life, like the music for different scenes in a film. The resulting music had a greater emotional resonance than she was able to convey through her communication device, and she felt heard. The last song lyrics Aubrey wrote before she was discharged ended with "hopeful...brighter...." I could only hope that she would have access to more counseling after she left the hospital.

Whenever I worked with a patient like that Aubrey, I was grateful for the counseling education that had been a part of my graduate music therapy degree. Knowing how to listen and reflect, either with words or with music, and to respect patients' feelings was critical in a therapeutic process that included music, because music often elicited direct emotional responses both positive and negative. Interestingly, patients who were active musicians prior to their injuries often were the least likely to want or respond to music therapy during their initial recovery. Being in a musical environment only reminded them of their losses. On the other hand, patients who were not musicians often found music to be the one avenue where they felt safe exploring their post-traumatic abilities and feelings.

I remember an 85 year-old man who refused all therapies after a stroke left him paralyzed on one side and unable to produce more than grunts. The largest of our aides could not get him out of his bed. When I went to his room and made a fool of myself singing and dancing for him, however, he began to tap his non-paralyzed foot under the covers and smile. A day later, he came to a music therapy group and when we used his grunt as the "oh" in his favorite hymn, *Oh, How I Love Jesus*, he responded by lengthening it ("Aaoooh") in subsequent choruses. Just that one improvement in his ability to interact seemed to give him hope and he began to attend all of his therapies the next day.

***

Melissa, a 15 year old, was brought to her music therapy session by one of the transport aides who gestured to tell me that today had been just as bad as the previous one. Melissa was in crisis. She had survived a traumatic brain injury and had been admitted to our rehabilitation hospital 10 days prior. She was incontinent, unable to speak independently due to aphasia, and paralyzed on her right side. (Aphasia is a disorder of language; any of a number of problems with conceptualizing thoughts and forming them into words, phrases, sentences.) After a couple of days in which she became more alert and aware of herself, she became increasingly more depressed and now she had stopped participating in therapy and stopped eating or drinking. She pulled out the first IV they gave her for fluids; the IV was now inserted into the back of her left hand. With her right hand paralyzed, there was nothing she could do about it. As a younger survivor, Melissa had a chance to gain back significant skills, but she needed to be working and she needed sustenance. The medical team would soon have to insert a feeding tube in order to give her nutrients.

Melissa was referred to music therapy because of her age, her need for communication work, and the team's hope that getting engaged with her favorite music might motivate her. I already had advice from her physical therapist, occupational therapist, and speech-language pathologist on what I could work on if Melissa started to get involved in music therapy -- but up to this point, all she would do is glance at one of two cassette tapes I held up, perhaps indicating that she was making a choice. (Her family had told me about her favorite genres and artists.) She didn't respond at all to live music or the opportunity to play instruments. The right side of her face was sagging (part of the paralysis) so sometimes it was even difficult to tell if she was moving her gaze from one side to another.

On that day I started by moving through some live music; singing and playing with guitar, then keyboard -- and then, when Melissa didn't show any response, I laid her left hand on a deep, resonant drum and played it so she could feel the vibrations. She seemed completely detached. Finally, I moved to the cabinet and pulled out two cassettes, holding them up to her at eye level.

"Ok…let's just listen to some music then. Which of these two would you like?" I asked.

Her gaze lingered a bit longer on a "greatest hits" tape from Cher. I put it in and sat back as we listened to *If I Could Turn Back Time*. Melissa did not respond in any significant way, but she stayed alert and kept her eyes on the cassette player and cassette cover, which I had placed on a music stand in front of her. As the song played on, I scanned the selections from the tape and saw another that made the radio playlists the previous year: *After All*. When the first selection concluded, I forwarded the tape to that song and pushed play.

Almost as soon as the song began, a change came over Melissa. She straightened up in her wheelchair and began looking at me as well as the player and tape cover. And, as the chorus began, she fixed her eyes on me. The distortion of her face seemed to fade into natural symmetry and I felt as if I was seeing the girl as she would have appeared before the brain injury. Afterwards, I would struggle to explain this perception in my documentation, but it was there. We stared at each other as the song continued and suddenly, Melissa spoke. "I remember," she whispered clearly, "I remember." Tears began to flow down her face.

I took her left hand in mine, avoiding the IV. "You remember hearing this song?" She nodded yes. Her face returned, in my eyes, to its previous uneven state, but she was still engaged with me. "And maybe you were with friends when it was playing?" She nodded yes again, with a lopsided smile.

There was a knock on the door. The transport aide had arrived to take Melissa to her next session in the speech therapy wing. "I'm so glad we listened to this today," I told her, wiping her tears gently with a tissue. "Come back on Tuesday and we'll do it again." I couldn't follow her. My next patient was waiting.

Afterwards, I thought about what happened. It occurred to me that perhaps, after becoming conscious after the brain injury, Melissa had been unable to recognize herself. Maybe the neural network that connected her to her memories was disrupted and she found herself in an unfamiliar body in an unfamiliar place, unable to communicate and ask questions that might help her find out what happened. In that situation, wouldn't many of us give up? Perhaps, like many of us, she also had a song or two that was inexorably tied to good memories, good friends, happy times. And maybe that song, in this instance, connected the dots.

Later that afternoon, Melissa's speech therapist appeared in my doorway. "What happened with Melissa in music therapy today?" she asked. I immediately wondered if something was wrong. Perhaps the session was too upsetting for her. "What do you mean?" I asked.

"Melissa did wonderfully in speech today," the therapist reported excitedly. "She worked on everything I gave her. And when I checked with nursing just now? She drank her nutrition drink!"

Sure enough, the next day brought more good news. Melissa had begun to participate in therapy again, and to accept some food and water. When she returned to music therapy the day after that, we leapfrogged over the music listening and began to write the first of several songs she would compose during her stay. Music therapy was, indeed, an outlet for her --- though there was never again as powerful a moment as the one when the wall between Melissa's past and present came tumbling down.

***

John was 32 years old and an air-conditioning repairman. One hot summer day, for reasons no one ever figured out, he fell off the flat roof of a strip shopping center to the pavement below and suffered a traumatic brain injury. He survived but was unable to walk, and there were more serious problems as well.

When I met John at our rehabilitation hospital, his memory for events surrounding the accident was gone, and his memory for things day-to-day at the hospital was patchy. More importantly, John had lost the ability to understand spoken and written language. He could respond to simple gestures (the invitation to a handshake, for example), but it seemed that he heard our words as just a series of nonsense syllables, or at best, mixed-up words. What made communication even more difficult is that his own speech, once out of his mouth, was also gibberish to him -- and while John could speak clearly he sometimes used the wrong word or mangled his sentence structure. "Get in the broom," he said to his occupational therapist, requesting a hairbrush and assuming his instructions were clear. When the OT failed to produce a brush, John repeated his muddled request and eventually became aggravated to the point of anger, shoving the therapist away and refusing to cooperate with any activity.

John had a type of receptive aphasia. Among the areas damaged by his injury was a small region in the left hemisphere of his brain, behind the ear. John's doctor and treatment team referred him to music therapy because his family had said he had some musical background. The team hoped that having a successful experience would lessen John's overall level of frustration and perhaps encourage him to participate in his therapy program.

In reviewing John's medical chart, I discovered that he was a substitute organist at his Presbyterian church and I wondered if perhaps it would be best to avoid words altogether in our first session. Therefore, when the aide pushed John's wheelchair through my door on Thursday afternoon, I was waiting with my electronic piano keyboard set to the "pipe organ" sound.

John was tall, thin and pale, but his handshake was firm and he looked at me directly, perhaps bracing himself for yet another onslaught of unintelligible babble. I smiled at him but didn't speak; instead, I simply wheeled him up to the electronic piano, and sat down on his left. Tapping him under his left arm, I gestured for him to put his hands on the keys. At the first sound of the "organ," John shifted in his wheelchair, sat up taller, and arranged his fingers. He immediately began playing the Doxology: music familiar to most Protestant congregations -- usually played after the offering.

Each beat required him to accurately play at least two notes with his left hand and three with his right. He played confidently. On the sixth beat, John missed a note in his right hand -- and instantly corrected it. I stifled a gasp at this clear music comprehension. Playing the second phrase, he stopped and backed up, repeating two beats when he made another error. He could, it seemed, listen, understand, and correct music in a way that he couldn't with language. I had read a case study in which this happened, but had never seen it in person.

As John finished the Doxology, I looked at him, expecting to see a smile or other acknowledgement of his accomplishment. Instead, he just looked intently at his fingers, as if waiting for them to begin playing again. After a few seconds, I reached across him and played the first few notes of a frequently chosen Protestant hymn, *Holy, Holy, Holy.*

Within the first six notes, John replaced my hand with his and took over. He played the entire hymn, using both hands, and I began to sing along -- quietly at first, so that he wouldn't feel forced to keep up a tempo, then more loudly as I saw that he was confident. At the end of the third verse (the last for which I could recall the words) I slowed down, indicating that the hymn should end. John picked up this cue (more comprehension) and provided the traditional organ conclusion, including the "Amen." We smiled at each other as any two musicians would after a successful duet, and I started us off on our next hymn. John continued to correct his mistakes and respond to my singing, demonstrating the ability to hear, evaluate and modify his musical expression.

The aide returned at the end of our thirty minute session. John and I had yet to speak a word to each other. As I unlocked the brakes of his wheelchair and pulled him away from the keyboard toward the door, I smiled at him and said -- with what I hoped was enough inflection and facial expression to get the meaning across -- "Thank you, John. That was fun!" John reached out for my hand and when I gave it to him, he put it between both of his and gripped it tightly, pulling me towards him. His eyes were full of tears and his voice shook as he said, "Thank you," and then:

"My leaf is in your hands."

I was excited about what John had shown me in the session. His ability to play familiar, well-rehearsed hymns on the piano might have been explained as an automatic behavior, a kind of "muscle memory." But John was able to stop and correct himself and this demonstrated that he had some conscious, deliberate control over his movements and, more interestingly, comprehension of musical input that was better than his comprehension of language input. I hoped this meant that he could learn and play new music, but to do that, he would have to be able to read music. I knew from his speech therapist that he could not read words. Would music be different?

The rehab team's prediction about music therapy proved to be right. After our first sessions, John was more cooperative with his therapists, nurses, and aides. He broke new ground in music therapy, as well. In our second week of sessions, John began to initiate some playing on his own, without waiting for me to suggest a song or hymn. One day he fingered a descending line of notes that sounded familiar to me, and I gestured to him, hoping he would play it again. He did, and after a moment, I realized that it was the old standard, *Fly Me to the Moon.* I pulled one of my music books off the shelf, found the song, and placed the open book on the stand at the back of the keyboard. John peered at it, seeming confused, and I pointed to the first note of the song. He put his index finger next to mine and looked at me, saying, "What?"

I reached across him and pushed the key for the first note
with one hand, my other hand still pointing at the music
book. He looked from one to the other, put his right hand
over mine and took over the melody, this time
continuing it beyond the first phrase as he followed the
printed music in the fake book. Was he reading the
music? During the initial part of the song, which he had
been playing by memory, he played quickly and seemed
to be using both his ear and eyes. Later on, however, in a
part he had not been able to remember, he was obviously
using the book.

I left him playing and walked quickly down the hall to
get the director of the speech-language pathology
program who was also John's speech therapist. She
followed me back to my office and watched as John
continued to have little trouble reading melodies from
the pages in front of him. When I turned the pages to
another song, we noticed that once again I had to show
him the first note on the keyboard before he could start.
Suddenly we both realized what was happening. John
was not reading symbolically. He was reading spatially.

Anyone who has taken a music lesson probably learned
the notes of the treble clef: F-A-C-E for the spaces and E-
G-B-D-F ("Every Good Boy Does Fine") for the lines. We
learn to match each note to a string or fingering on our
instrument, like the C on the piano. As we play, we pick
out the notes somewhat like we pick out letters and
sounds when we learn to read. Soon, however, we start
to recognize the "shape" of music. We see a descending

series of notes and we don't think about each individual one ("first I play a C, then that's a B, and after that an A...") but simply recognize that each note is one below the one before it, and move our fingers accordingly. Soon we learn to recognize the space between notes that are separated, and what an octave (8 notes apart) looks like. At some point, the only note we may identify symbolically, by its letter name and location on the music, is the first one. Every note after that is just a recognizable distance moving up or down.

As I soon confirmed, John could not identify notes by letter name. If I asked him to "play a C," my words were, as usual for him, confusing. If I wrote a single note on a page and showed it to him, he could not identify or play it. The title of a song, printed on the page had no meaning. However, if I showed him a written melody and pointed out the first note of the song on the piano, he could play it; and if it was a song he knew before his injury, he smiled as soon as he recognized it. Although John's ability to read or understand speech did not return at all during his rehabilitation hospital stay, he regained more and more of his skill for reading music and refining his playing through listening and correcting his own mistakes.

This was 1993 and the research on neurological pathways for language and music was not yet exploding as it would when researchers gained ready access to various brain imaging techniques. But John had shown me what science would eventually confirm: that some activities of music-making have their own neurological pathways that may be preserved when language functions are lost. Like many of us who worked in neurological rehabilitation, I had a chance to see a phenomenon first-hand that would later be confirmed in published research. More than that, I was grateful that music therapy had given John a way to communicate, and to ensure that music remained a part of his life.

INTERLUDE

How Did I Get Here?

I grew up in a home filled with music. My parents were fans of jazz, and they played jazz recordings throughout my childhood. My maternal grandmother played stride piano by ear, and my mother had studied formally through college. At my parents' parties it wasn't unusual for someone to sit down at the piano and lead other guests in singing American standards: Gershwin, Cole Porter, tunes from Broadway. My mother also loved classical music and the classical music radio station was on daily. We had wonderful children's records, too, with music from around the world. My younger brother's and my ears were filled with music from the time we were born -- and before.

Listening to classical music made me aware the rules of balance and harmony and form as well as all the interesting ways the rules can be broken. Listening to jazz and its improvisation helped me learn how to follow the harmony of a piece even when the melody disappeared, and how to keep track of the beat even when the music was highly complex. Listening to the standards of the American Songbook made me appreciate a sophisticated interplay of lyrics and melody. Of course, I didn't know I was learning any of that; I was just growing up with music all around me.

We lived in a suburb north of Chicago and its school district was one of the first in the country to adopt the Suzuki violin method. My own experience as a music student started with group violin lessons the summer after first grade. When I showed an aptitude for it, my parents started me on private lessons. Although the mothers in our group did not learn the violin as the Japanese mothers did, our Suzuki experience was otherwise consistent with its philosophy: we learned violin as children learn other things, through play and listening and watching. Before we ever bowed a note, we played games to become comfortable with holding our instruments: shaking hands and waving as we held our violins under our chins, and imitating windshield washers with our bows. By the time we began to learn repertoire, holding the violin and bow were second nature. We also learned to play with distractions, like a feather tickling our noses.

Most importantly, we played by ear. As prescribed by the program, my mother played the recordings of all the music at home so every melody was familiar before I ever started playing it. All this meant that as I entered fourth grade -- a time when some school districts introduce violin study for the first time -- I already had a solid foundation of comfort with my instrument and was already playing simple sonata movements by memory.

When I began to play more advanced pieces, I did not have to worry about what my body was doing, and because I had started listening at an early age, I had a "good ear" for playing in tune. As anyone who has listened to young people playing instruments can attest, playing in tune is a valuable skill!

Being part of an early American Suzuki program was special and it shaped my identity as "a violinist," in the same way other children with focused interests might identify as "gymnasts" or "ballet students". Students and teachers from Japan visited every other year and there was always media coverage of their arrival at the airport with all of us playing our violins at the gate, and interviews with us on the local news. Each visit featured a workshop where we played with the Japanese students (all of whom were more advanced than we were at the same age) and learned from their teachers. Mr. Honda, a senior teacher from Japan, would test us in all sorts of fun ways. When several of us had learned both parts to Bach's Concerto for Two Violins, for example, he divided all of the American and Japanese students who could play it into two groups on the stage where we were working. We began playing and then, one at a time, Mr. Honda would tug on a student's ear and guide him or her, still playing, across to the other side. When the student passed the invisible center line, he or she would switch parts without stopping. Sometimes he would tug us back and forth across the line so that we switched parts every few measures. That level of comfort and fun with playing, I know now, was something I would seek in all my future musical experiences.

As I became more involved in violin playing, my identity transitioned from "a violinist" to "a very good violinist." The struggles everyone has in junior high were softened a bit for me by having a home in the orchestra room, and by having like-minded peers at weekend lessons in theory, solfege, and chamber music at our area's community music school. The chamber music, in particular, was a huge influence on me. As I learned to be part of a quartet (two violins, viola, and 'cello) I was learning to listen more intently and to play with more variation. In many chamber music pieces, you play one moment in unison with the other violinist, then the next with the cellist, and then you are a soloist as the others accompany you. You have to divide your attention and yet listen to the whole at the same time. What wonderful practice for observing, making decisions, and playing in a music therapy session!

I spent several weeks each summer at music camps and festivals starting when I was 12 years old and continuing through high school. Just like any other camp experience, I arrived scared and left reluctantly -- but these summer music experiences on college campuses were not about games and activities: they were intensive work intended to train us for music careers. I was successful, always placing at the front of the violin sections, often as the concertmaster, and that reinforced the idea that I was on the right path. At home during the school year, I played at school, on the weekends, and at special events. I practiced before school, after school, and built a repertoire of solo, orchestral and chamber music pieces. I occasionally won awards and got a write-up in the local news; the story was always that I would go on to study and perform as a violinist.

Except...there was something else. Somehow, I had heard about music therapy. The idea of it was potent enough that I remember my mother and me looking to see which colleges offered a music therapy degree. Friends from high school tell me now that I often spoke about it as a career or avocation, and I told an interviewer that I wanted to (in the terminology of the day) "use music to help mentally retarded children." Yet by the time I was choosing colleges and preparing audition materials, all my focus was on a violin performance degree. I had spent nine years preparing, after all. I had the opportunity for full scholarships, and I loved being a top violinist.

In the end, I chose the University of Cincinnati College-Conservatory of Music, primarily because after a special audition, I was offered the opportunity to study with one of the pre-eminent coaches in the country, Dorothy DeLay. She came to "CCM" every two weeks from her home base at Julliard in New York City to teach 6 of us who had been chosen for the program. It was a heady time and it was all about violin. I was in an assigned chamber music group and also played in a second one that was created to perform around the city. I studied with Miss DeLay and was part of a group of exceptional players. I played in the orchestra and a baroque music group, and spent hours in the practice rooms. My roommate was a music student, most of my friends were music students, and I can't remember anyone ever speaking to me about a class outside the conservatory (though I know I took some, as required by the university). I began to make plans for a career as a chamber musician: a member of a professional quartet.

Except…I kept hearing about music therapy, and the idea nagged at me. Like many young adults, I was learning to think in broader terms about where I fit into the world. I was exploring my own spirituality. As each semester of college passed, I felt a little less comfortable in focusing solely on the violin and a little more curious about what else I could accomplish as a musician. I felt as if I were neglecting parts of myself in order to fit into a specific, narrow world.

My family had embraced a variety of music, but my parents were also avid readers and concerned citizens. They made sure my brother and I were aware of circumstances outside our safe, suburban environment, and there were few dinners at our home that did not involve discussion of a newspaper article, debate over a political issue, or answering a question by pulling out a volume of the encyclopedia, a dictionary, or an atlas. I was curious about medicine, psychology, sociology, how children learn, how the brain works, how to address poverty and racism. For me, a violin performance degree left little time to think or learn about any of that, and as far as I could tell, no one saw that as a problem. Even a related field like music education wasn't valued at the conservatory; at our juries each year (basically the "final exam" for music majors) the panel responded to a passing solo with "thank you," and a less successful one with "have you considered a music education degree?" as if music education was only for those who couldn't succeed as performers.

Meanwhile, I knew in my heart of hearts that I had a different comfort level with performing than my peers, especially those in Miss DeLay's elite studio. I began to feel that I had reached a pinnacle in my playing; while the other DeLay students were mastering the next Paganini caprice for the excitement of demonstrating technical prowess, I felt happiness in learning only certain pieces: music that spoke to me and satisfied me in some deeper way. And I had developed a right hand shake that at the time, I attributed to nerves, though I learned later that I, like women on my mother's side of the family, had an inherited tremor. There were times when playing the violin was joy itself, but there were times when I wondered what I was working towards.

Then, one day at the beginning of my junior year, I ran into a graduate student I barely knew (but to whom I must have spoken about my interests) and she told me she had found out about an "Introduction to Music Therapy" class at a nearby college. Did I want to take it with her? It seemed like fate. We signed up and began driving there one evening a week.

It was the first step and I never turned back. After researching the requirements for music therapy students, I began taking classes outside the conservatory that would allow me to enter one of the "master's-equivalency" music therapy degree programs around the country. (These programs get you caught up on music therapy coursework you didn't take as an undergraduate and merge that into master's degree work.)

Then I began to tell everyone what I was planning. It was a difficult time, to say the least. Important people in my life thought it was a terrible mistake and told me I was going through a phase, or not thinking clearly, or squandering the gift God had given me. I felt support from only a few people -- and one of them, my future husband (an engineering student) didn't really understand the implications of the choice. I myself was unprepared for the impact of moving forward from the single identity I had developed as "the very good violinist."

Fortunately, one of the very few people who did understand and who encouraged me was Miss DeLay. She told me that she had once considered a career in psychiatry (something I confirmed when I read her biography) and that she understood my fascination with learning how music affects and changes people. As my junior year ended, she did two critically important things for me. First, she made sure I was accepted into an exclusive summer quartet program where I could have an intensive chamber music experience: a kind of "farewell" to highly concentrated study in my favorite area of performance. Then, she helped me schedule an early senior recital and fill it with repertoire that would be emotionally satisfying while meeting the requirements of the conservatory. I successfully completed that recital in November and after that, never played another note in our lessons. Instead, with her encouragement, I spent each lesson talking with her about what new discovery I'd made in my music therapy class, or anatomy & physiology, or abnormal psychology.

Three years later, when I finished my master's degree, I wrote Miss DeLay to thank her. Though she was a renowned teacher, she had a justified reputation as someone who was scatter-brained about certain details, including her students' names, and I did not expect her to remember me. It was a lovely surprise when she wrote back and retold stories about our music therapy discussions from that last year.

Many of the music therapy students I teach today did not have the background I was fortunate to have. Many are still working to master musical skills as they begin studying all the other aspects of a degree in healthcare and therapy. Their desire is just as strong as mine, but their public schools have diminished music education programming and their families haven't had the resources to help them study privately. Furthermore, their music training seems to emphasize the acquisition of repertoire over solid preparation in technique and ear training. Many of the music therapy students at my college must work on strengthening their internal pulse, learning accompaniments in multiple genres, and being able to respond musically moment-by-moment -- all at the same time they must focus on psychology, research methods, and music therapy. I wish they all could have a level of mastery in music before they begin music therapy study, because that foundation is both critical to our clients and just the beginning of what they need to learn.

CHAPTER FOUR

A Day in Special Education – Part I

Many people first hear about music therapy through experiences with special education. Many have read stories about how music therapy helps children on the autism spectrum or children with communication or behavior challenges. Music therapy became more available to children in public school special education because of the passage of the Individuals with Disabilities Act in 1997 and its definition of "related services." Related services are interventions, like physical therapy, or music therapy, that are shown to be necessary for a child to achieve the goals written by his team for his individualized education plan (IEP). If an assessment shows that a service is necessary, the school district is required to provide it and pay for it.

Once music therapy was confirmed to be a related service by the federal Office of Special Education, an increasing number of parents requested assessments for their children. Some school districts, recognizing that music therapy was beneficial for most students in certain programs (early childhood, autism), simply hired MT-BCs to provide music therapy to all of them, saving pricier individual assessments for students outside those programs. In this and other ways, via federal, state and local funding, music therapy became a regular part of public school special education in many districts. This chapter and the next are about what was, for me, a typical day as a contracted music therapist for a large, diverse suburban school district.

October
Tarrant County, Texas
Morning

I headed out to my car to start the busiest day of my week as a music therapist for a school district in north Texas. I loaded my guitar into the back seat and then checked the trunk to be sure I had everything properly packed: my box of session files and visual aids, my boxes of instruments, a foldable music stand, and cloth bags to carry whatever I would need into each school. Finally I put my tote into the passenger seat after checking to see that I had the clipboard and charts I would need to collect data. I would be doing 6 sessions at 4 different schools with clients ranging in age from 3 to 16. By the end of the afternoon, I would have seen 28 students in scheduled sessions, conducted one assessment, and -- though I didn't know it yet -- had an impromptu musical interaction that would start with a student's meltdown.

It would be a busy day, but I was aware how fortunate I was that those of us doing special education work no longer kept the kinds of schedules our predecessors maintained. As an intern, I spent a day a week with a music therapist in a school district where she did eight sessions in five different schools in just six hours. We ate lunch in 10 minutes standing in a parking lot and consulted with teachers in the hallways. There was never a moment in which we weren't in motion. I used to get a headache in the morning as I waited for her to pick me up, and I didn't have to do what she did: plan and practice and create in the evenings at home.

At some point in the intervening years, the music therapists in our area began networking, sharing ideas, and most importantly, talking about contracts and rates openly. This transparency helped everyone negotiate more realistic job descriptions and parameters. By the time I took this school district job, the pay was reasonable and the workload busy but manageable.

***

8:00 am: My first stop of the day was the local post office, where I always stopped and did something: mailed a music therapy brochure, copied some music, or bought some supplies. This was an important trip for my tax return: the IRS did not allow me to deduct the first trip of my day and the drive to the school district was the longest one. If I went straight there, I wouldn't be able to deduct that mileage. Like any self-employed business woman, I needed to know tax law in addition to all the other skills for my job.

***

8:25 am: I arrived at my first school for a once-a-month session with an early childhood special education class. My role here was as a consultant. Every month I ran a session with seven little ones, ages 3-5, and showed the teacher and aides how they could do a similar group for the rest of the month. Each week I visited a different classroom. I created activities that would reinforce the year-long goals for the class: communication, behavior, and socialization, as well as highlighting the time of year and any holiday themes. Because the teacher and aides couldn't accompany themselves on guitar or piano, I recorded some songs and designed others to be done with just rhythmic beats from clapping or drums.

Teachers have many musical resources. Some are musicians themselves. There are wonderful children's song recordings by talented, creative artists. There are books of "piggyback" song lyrics: academic concepts that can be sung to familiar tunes. It's now common to have software programs which allow children to create their own music. So my purpose in coming to this class was not just to bring music; it was to show how being both targeted and flexible with the music could help the individual children with their individual needs. At this session I demonstrated how pauses in the music would help Brad maintain attention without any other reminders, and how Keshawn spoke up more when we slowly chanted three key words, rather than singing them. As I sang a letter identification song, I pointed out to the teacher (in the pauses between verses, as I kept the guitar accompaniment going) how the letter names occurred on the downbeats of measures -- and I showed her how the melody lines that led up to them created a tension that Sari responded to by leaning forward and trying to be the first to say the letter name.

I knew that the teacher and her aides, all great people, would do their best to replicate the things I demonstrated. The district only paid for one consult session per month, so we had to make it work as well as we could. At 9:05, I finished up and wrote some documentation in the hallway outside the class. By 9:15, I was back in my car and on my way to my second stop of the day.

***

9:30 am: The students in the middle school classroom saw me once a week. They all had intellectual disabilities but were able to participate in a traditional classroom set-up, all sitting at desks and learning together with one teacher. It was unusual for me to see students in a class like this because funds were limited and the music therapist was usually assigned to work with the students who had more significant challenges with a school setting. The principal of this school, however, was an advocate for music therapy and she had always been successful in scheduling this once-a-week session. There were 12 students in the class and the teacher and I used my time to encourage them to be creative and give them a chance to work together as a team. These were skills that might have been neglected while everyone focused on basic academic skills. We also worked on sequencing and memory with songs and instruments. Then, near the end of the session, we worked on audiation.

Audiation is what you do when you "hear" something without any actual sound being present. Imagine the melody to the national anthem. You can "hear" each note, even though no one is singing. Audiation is also part of holding something in working memory, like a phone number or an instruction. I had been reading some theories about audiation and children with intellectual disabilities like Down syndrome. One theory was that a lack of ability to audiate might explain why these children had trouble following multiple-step directions or connecting two pieces of information.

So, at the end of this session, I took a familiar folk song that we sang with verses and a chorus and got everyone singing.

When I first came to this land
I was not a wealthy man
But the land was sweet and good -- and
I did what I could.

I led this song in a lively way, though moderating the tempo occasionally so everyone could keep up. The dancing style led me to end each chorus with an exclamation:

But the land was sweet and good -- and
I did what I could – HEY!

As a musician, that last shout seemed natural, even though it's not in the original lyrics. I couldn't help it, and it was fun to see how much the students enjoyed getting to the end, throwing their arms in the air and shouting, "HEY!" Even better, the shout allowed us all to test the students' ability to audiate, because by the third chorus, I went silent, miming my guitar playing and articulating the lyrics without a voice. The students, who had learned what to do, followed along with their eyes and "inner voice" -- and only when I finished mouthing the last line did they raise their arms in the air and shout, "HEY!"

We would have opportunities to increase the challenge in future sessions, but it was time to go. I documented the session, packed up the car again, and headed off to school #3.

***

10:30 am: My job at the next school was to complete an assessment with a 7 year old boy named Peter, to see if music therapy should be added to his IEP: the individual educational plan developed for every special education student. In this school district, the administration was voluntarily offering music therapy services to students with severe intellectual disabilities, autism, and classes like the ones I had seen, without requiring an individual "eligibility" assessment. Peter, however, didn't fall into

73

those categories; he attended regular education classes with just some support from a resource teacher and speech therapist. There were some students like this who responded so strongly to music therapy in an assessment that it was added to their IEP as a related service. Peter's parents hoped I would tell the district that Peter was one of those students. Peter had a mild hearing impairment, some problems with his speech articulation, and his education team wanted him to increase his attention span.

In any public school special education eligibility assessment, a music therapist has to answer the question, "is music therapy required for this student to benefit from his program?" The assessment process can seem a bit callous because we think: shouldn't every child with special needs have music if they enjoy it? The answer to that is, of course, yes -- but here again, music therapy is different. Music for enrichment and enjoyment was readily available. In Peter's case, his school brought in volunteers to perform and share songs. Teachers could play recordings or even play music themselves in a classroom, and Peter attended music education class with his peers twice a week. None of this was an added expense for the school district. Music therapy, however -- like other therapies -- would be specially designed for Peter, and would have to be provided on a schedule that would best help him achieve his goals. That was an expense, and if the money was spent on Peter, it couldn't be spent elsewhere for another student.

That's why the assessment process I was using was regimented and why a colleague and I were working on formalizing it. (See the Interlude after Chapter 5 for more about this.) I had spent time over the past week reviewing paperwork and doing interviews and observations. Now it was time to do the music therapy session I'd designed based on all that and see how Peter would respond. I would collect data and compare it to my observations of Peter working without music therapy. I also knew that if I wanted to see how Peter would respond to music therapy over time, this assessment session couldn't feel like a checklist. It needed to be musical and spontaneous and fun. I had things I needed to watch for and document, but I also needed to involve Peter as I would in any session.

Peter was eager to play the instruments I had with me, and he swayed back and forth to the music, smiling. There was no difference, however, in the way he approached education tasks or how long he paid attention to schoolwork. In other words, his enjoyment didn't translate into motivation or assistance in working on his IEP goals. In private therapy, his pleasure would have been enough for us to get started and we could let the musical experiences gradually build a therapeutic relationship and important skills, but here, in this financial environment, I needed to see signs that music therapy would have an impact on school goals within the next semester. And at this point, Peter just liked listening to the music. The report I wrote would note that music therapy was not required for Peter, but that Peter should have as many chances to participate in musical activities as possible. I knew his parents would be disappointed, but I felt confident about my decision based on the data I had and the requirements of the law.

I didn't have time to write many notes right at that moment, though, so as I drove to the next school, I dictated my observations and data into a small tape recorder. "Onward!" I said to myself. If I didn't run into traffic, I might be able to sit down for a short lunch break at my next school.

***

11:30 am: I arrived at my "home school:" the elementary school where any mail came to me and where I did a majority of my weekly sessions. Every student in its two self-contained classrooms had significant intellectual, communication and behavior or social challenges and all had music therapy written into their IEPs. I had made good time, so I headed towards the teacher's lounge, thinking I might even have a chance to chat with…

Uh oh. As I walked in the front door, I heard screaming from the cafeteria to my right. As I looked in, I immediately saw Aaron, a short thin boy on the autism spectrum, 8 years old; he was standing on top of his class' lunch table, crying and screaming and throwing pieces of bread. His teacher, Pam, and her aide, Sue, were balancing their attempts to calm Aaron with their efforts to keep the rest of the class from joining the melee. They needed some help. I stepped up to the table and swung my guitar case up in the air on one side and my bag of materials up on the other. "Hey, Aaron!" I said, as normally as possible, and then kind of sing-songed the question: "want to go make some music?"

I shifted my bag to the one also holding my guitar so I could reach a hand out towards Aaron. To everyone's relief, he turned and got down off the table, moving toward me. I quickly asked if it would be okay to take him out of the room, then immediately started a marching song. Aaron gently took my pinkie between two of his fingers: his version of holding hands.

We're walking, we're walking
Through the hall, through the school
We're walking, we're walking
We can march and walk."

The lyrics were ridiculously simple and a little too young for Aaron, but I couldn't get my brain to come up with anything more interesting. I tried adding a little spice to the melody while marching more or less in place until I saw where Aaron wanted to go. He led me, quite deliberately, forward then right into a hallway, then right again, then left. He knew exactly where he wanted to go and soon we were in front of the music room, where I conducted sessions on the days when the music teacher wasn't there. I quickly unlocked the door and opened it, keeping up my musical narration as we entered. I had no sooner dropped my bag on the floor than Aaron got into it. He pulled out a file folder that had been transformed into a visual aid for a song he liked; it had colorful laminated pieces on it that could be moved around and attached to the folder with hook-and-loop fasteners. He walked it over to the music stand, placed the folder on the stand and promptly sat down in the chair next to the stand, looking at me expectantly.

I recognized my cue and, giving thanks for my always-in-tune guitar, I pulled it out as fast as I could, starting to sing the reggae song that went with the file folder before the guitar was in my lap.

Six little fish, swimming up and down;
Six little fish in my blue pond;
Close my eyes and what do I see?

I put my hand in front of my eyes and Aaron, as he would in a regular session, pulled one of the laminated fish off the file folder "pond." I sang again:

Five little fish are looking at me --- let's count!

Aaron had already joined me for "Let's count!" and now he chanted the number sequence with me as I pointed to the fish. "One, two, three, four, five. How many? Five!"

We worked our way down to "no more fishes" and finished the song. Aaron, now with no sign of the anxiety he showed earlier, leapt off the chair and headed for the door.

"But what about the goodbye song?" I asked, and immediately Aaron pivoted, came back to the chair and sat down. We sang the simple goodbye song that ended our regular sessions: I offered "good..." and Aaron finished "bye!"

I raced after Aaron, who pretty much skipped to his classroom, where everyone had returned from lunch. Aaron's teacher and I talked quickly, and I learned that one of the regular side dishes for lunch had not been available, and that Aaron hadn't been able to understand its absence or anyone's explanations. This led to the meltdown -- and also explained why Aaron had appreciated being able to find a place where things went as expected and hadn't changed. Music therapy can be a safe place.

I wondered if I had time to eat a banana.

CHAPTER FIVE

A Day in Special Education – Part II

Tarrant County
Afternoon

12:05 pm: I grabbed a banana and munched it as I quickly set up the music room for the three music therapy sessions I was running that afternoon. I carried most of what I needed with me, but I did use the nice solid music stand in the room to display visual aids. When I walked back to the hallway where the self-contained special education classrooms were located, I found one of the teachers, Dorothy, out in the hall bent over with laughter.

"What's going on?" I asked.

"Oh my gosh," she gasped, pointing back at the classroom. "Camille! I can't let her see me laughing!" As I looked through the door, I could see Camille, an eight-year old girl who had developmental disabilities and had recently suffered a stroke. Despite these challenges, Camille was a cheerful girl who loved to give hugs and who worked hard. She was in her "standing box," a large wooden frame with a desk platform at chest height.

These frames are important for people who cannot stand on their own, because weight-bearing through the legs helps prevent contractures and improves circulation. They can be, however, difficult to get into, and Colleen needed two or three people to get her stretched out and secured into the straps, her arms on the desk. It was also a painful procedure.

"What happened with Camille?" I asked. "Is she okay?"

"Oh, she's just fine!" Dorothy replied cryptically. "You know how her family only speaks Spanish at home, right? And how the aphasia has kept her from doing much more than repeating 'hi' and 'bye'?" I nodded. "So you wouldn't expect her to say much more in English, right?"

"Ok..." I said, waiting for the punch line.

"Well, we were just now getting her into the standing box and, poor dear, it was really hard today. I felt so bad for her. She was crying and Claire and Sue from next door were getting the straps set and extending her legs, and I was up top, talking to her and trying to keep her calm."

I nodded. I had seen this drama unfold before.

"And just as Sue got the last strap fixed in place, Camille took a deep breath, leaned towards me, and shouted, "F-you!" Dorothy started laughing again.

"No way!"

"Yes!" she said. "I had to run out here so she wouldn't see me crack up!"

We both laughed.

"Ok," I said, "while we're on the subject, let me tell you one. You know the instrument song I wrote -- the one that asks "What instrument will you pick today? What instrument will you pick today?" I sang the lines of the chorus.

"Sure," Dorothy said. She had a recording of it for use in her classroom.

"Well I was over at Greene Elementary the other day with this class of five kids. One of them, Jeremy..."

"Is that the Jeremy who used to be in Pam's class here?"

"Yes! That's him. So you know he loves singing, even if he mixes up the words."

"Sure."

"Ok, so I was over at Greene and we were doing that song. And suddenly I noticed that Jeremy was singing along, really enthusiastically, big smile on his face, swaying back and forth. Except what he was singing was, 'what instrument will you f--- today?' and he was giving me the finger!"

"What???"

"Yes! He wasn't doing it to be naughty -- he really somehow thought those were the words! I almost fell off my chair."

"What did you do?"

"Not a thing. I didn't want to bring attention to it." I shook my head. "But as you can imagine, I'm changing the words. We'll do 'what instrument will you *choose* today' from now on!"

***

12:15 Claire helped me take the first of three groups to music therapy. I marveled again at the good humor and smart management skills the aides had. They were making ridiculously little money and they dealt with all the toileting and dressing and feeding; a much more difficult job, really, than anyone's. And our special ed teachers! They had up to 8 children with significant disabilities in their classrooms, each with a completely distinct diagnosis, set of skills, set of challenges, and favorite type of praise. Each one required one-on-one attention and assistance, but the teacher and an aide did it all. They were extraordinary.

Each of my music therapy groups had three or four students in it, grouped according to ability levels and goals. There were three students in this group: Colleen, Philip, and Javier; they each had challenges that required lots of direct, individual work. Javier was 8 years old, on the autism spectrum, and a runner. If the music stopped for more than a second or two and I wasn't on alert, he'd be out of his chair and across the room, if not down the hall. So this group and every other group sat with their backs to the blackboard and me between them and the open room. I made sure Javier sat in the middle. I didn't want to have to stop him; I wanted the session and its set-up to help him succeed.

Colleen was a cherubic little girl, 8 years old, with multiple disabilities stemming from genetic disorders. She was termed "medically fragile" because of problems with breathing, and she had only one voluntary movement: the ability to tense and relax her right forearm. I used this to make her the most important musician in the room.

I had a switch: a large, round yellow button that could be pressed down to activate anything battery operated, or to play a recording made on the switch itself. For Colleen, I recorded the last word of one of our songs. If I slid this switch across Colleen's lap tray (the clear tray attached to her wheelchair) she could raise her right forearm and then, once the switch was underneath, relax her arm -- thereby pressing down on the switch. When we approached the end of the designated song, I slowed down and paused just before the final word, sliding the switch over to Colleen. The song couldn't end without her. Every time, when she put her arm down, heard the final word and heard me play the final chord, she lifted her head and beamed. She was a superstar!

Today, Colleen was having trouble relaxing her arm and it was already tensed up when I slid the switch over. We were finishing a song called *That Bear Makes Me Crazy* by Kevin Roth. In some classes, I had rewritten the words and used pictures to address a receptive language goal, but here we sang it as it was, just before the end of the session.

The song had a fun ending: "Oh, that bear makes me CRAAAAAZY!" Colleen's switch, of course, had "CRAZY!" recorded on it, so I always made a big deal about the lead-up and the harmonic cadence from my guitar just hanging there without the final word, note, and chord. (What if you sang "Happy Birthday" but, at the very end, stopped before "you"? That's the tension I'm describing.) On this day, as Colleen tried to relax and the tension of the cadence hung there, I felt my brain saying, "Finish the song!" -- and I wasn't the only one.

Philip was sitting to Colleen's right. Philip was a 9 year-old student on the autism spectrum; he didn't communicate verbally and followed directions only as part of familiar routines. He spent most of the day doing a repetitive motion that looked quite a bit like he was rowing invisible oars, very fast, at shoulder height. We suspected he did this as compensation for a sensory imbalance, and a sensory integration specialist from the occupational therapy program was working with him. Today, however, the movement was constant and Philip's head tilted to the right, away from Colleen. His eyes, as was often the case, didn't seem to focus on anything and he looked as though he wasn't listening to the music or paying attention to anything else in the room.

But when the pause in the "Bear" song became longer than usual, and my brain was straining for a resolution to the melody and harmony, Philip's arm movement suddenly stopped. He looked right at Colleen and threw his head back, rolling his eyes in what looked exactly like exasperation. With a heavy, audible sigh, he reached across her and hit the switch.

"CRAAAAAZY!" sang my recorded voice. I played the final chord and Colleen looked up and smiled.

Philip went back to rowing. He was satisfied. I was laughing. I love how music affects us!

***

12:45 pm: The second of the three sessions went well with students all showing progress. One of them, who did not show specific responses to music for two years in this group (and whom I'd therefore planned to dismiss at the end of the three-year reporting period), was suddenly responding specifically to the songs I'd used for two years. Not the new ones, just the ones that he'd had two years to process. He *was* responding, just in a very different time frame than most of us would. I was relieved my impatience hadn't cut off his therapy.

In fact, the only weak link in this particular session was me. I had deliberately written one of the songs with a C minor chord so I would have the chance to practice the bar chord on my guitar each time I used the song. On this day, most of what the students heard on that beat was a muddled mess. I needed to do some outside-the-session practicing, stat!

***

1:25 pm: When I went to the second classroom to pick up the three students for the final session, I found that two of them were absent. The only student present was Corey. I pondered what to do, because Corey had been the least responsive of the students in his group and I was anticipating that I would recommend removing music therapy from his IEP at the end of the year when his regular review came up. He wasn't responding with a long delay, like the student in the previous session. Music therapy just wasn't making a significant difference for him progressing towards his goals, which included interacting with others, maintaining attention on a task, and initiating requests.

Corey was 9 years old and nonverbal. He used a wheelchair and was hypotonic: one of the aides affectionately described him as "floppy." He could be sitting up one second and the next his head would be resting on his lap tray. He often flopped to the side, dangling one arm and letting his head tilt sideways. He would hold an item for a moment, and then drop it to the floor as his arm flopped down. A flop also signaled an interruption in his attention, so when he collapsed every other minute or so, he didn't stay engaged long enough to learn new things or develop relationships. For many of my students, specially chosen or constructed music was the one thing that kept them focused -- the one medium through which they communicated. Corey hadn't responded that way.

When Corey and I got to the music room, I decided to take him to the piano. With just the two of us, I thought, I could pull his wheelchair up next to my chair and perhaps get him involved with the keys and sounds. I removed his lap tray and pushed the wheelchair up to the lower end of the keyboard so his hands (if he took them off his lap) would easily rest on top of the keys. Maybe, I hoped, even if he didn't push the keys, he would respond to the vibrations of the piano as I played.

I told Corey I was going to get him started, and I took his dominant right hand and let it drop onto the lower keys. Several notes close together boomed out of the piano. I used both my hands and, without aiming at any particular notes, played a loud combination of notes from the upper register in response. Immediately, Corey lifted his right hand up and pushed it back down on the keys. It did not flop. He deliberately played another cluster of notes. I responded with another single beat of notes on my end of the keyboard. Then, Corey played two clusters in a row. Bum! Bum! I played a high note version: Bing! Bing! I looked over and Corey had turned his head and was looking directly at me with a huge smile. "Aaaah!" he exclaimed, then turned back to the piano and played two more clusters of notes.

Nothing about this cacophony would have sounded like music to anyone but us, but we were all that mattered. And frankly, we had a pretty regular rhythm going and the music didn't sound all that much different than that of the avant-garde composers whose premieres I had played at the conservatory. I varied my two "chords," playing one and then moving a ways higher to play the second one. Corey played his own cluster then reached up the keyboard to play his second, turning to grin at me as though saying, "Ha! Thought I'd miss that, did you? Joke's on you!"

After a few minutes of our improvised piece, Corey brought his left hand up to the piano. Corey rarely used his left hand and had never used it deliberately in music therapy, but now he had either decided he wanted to say more than he could with just the one hand or he was imitating me. Our joyful and dissonant music continued for another 5 minutes: an eternity in Coreyland. He had been more active and more eager to engage with me through facial expressions and vocalizations than he had in two and a half years.

Finally, he seemed to tire and, in a familiar movement, his head flopped forward. This time, however, his lap tray was gone and his head landed on the piano keys in front of him, playing a gentle cluster of notes as it descended. Still feeling the musical moment, I played a single gentle rejoinder. There was a pause...and then I saw Corey's head lift up slightly and descend, nodding twice so that now there were two gentle clusters that sounded out from the keys. Even in his tired state, he was still expressing himself and communicating with me.

What had happened?

Music therapy is not a single approach. Music therapists are creative, and as different as Mozart Symphony is from a Thelonious Monk improvisation, so are our musical interactions with clients. Music therapy sessions can be highly structured, to the point of a specific protocol that is repeated without variation: this can be helpful when conducting experimental research. In other approaches sessions are structured with a group of songs and musical pieces: the sessions have a similar arc, but the music within varies and the therapist may make on-the-spot changes to respond to or cue a client. This kind of session can be comforting, or help with focus, as it did for Aaron.

Another approach to music therapy sessions was developed by Paul Nordoff and Clive Robbins, and is therefore known by their names: Nordoff-Robbins Music Therapy. In this method, all of the music is created spontaneously in response to what the client brings to the session. Once a song is created or introduced it can be repeated, but the music therapist only does this when it is a natural response to the client's behavior or mood or interaction. Sessions are typically conducted by two music therapists: one at the piano or guitar, and one directly facing and interacting with the client or clients. The goal is to reach the musical being within every child; when that happens, the child will develop new abilities and behavior organically as a desire for deeper musical interactions and relationship develops.

Corey, at least in this one session, had a significant response to this improvisational type of music therapy. A couple of weeks later, I took some extra time to work with Corey at the piano again and he was just as enthusiastic as before. I reported on Corey's responses to the IEP team the following month, and we hoped that he would receive one-on-one sessions with me, but the request was not approved. Once again, it came down to funding. Although the "letter of the law" stated that Corey's extraordinary response to improvisational music -- which addressed his key educational goals -- should have resulted in his receiving individual sessions, the reality was that there was only so much money the district was going to spend on related services. In this district, that meant students would only be seen in groups. Corey's parents did not pursue the issue, so I attempted to include more spontaneous music opportunities in Corey's group sessions. It was not nearly as effective as one-on-one sessions would have been.

But on that particular afternoon, I didn't know the outcome. I drove home around 4pm, thrilled by Corey's response, disappointed in myself for not having tried something like this sooner. Relieved that I was there for Aaron. Determined to practice that C minor chord. Curious to do some more research on audiation. Tired. Satisfied.

INTERLUDE

Lifelong Learning

It's flattering to be viewed as an expert in something. It's also scary and a little ridiculous. There's always so much more to learn.

For several years in the mid-to-late 1990's I did quite a bit of traveling as a music therapy consultant. I had always imagined that it would be fun to be paid to travel a bit, stay in nice hotels, and get to talk about a subject I loved -- so when I got the chance to be a speaker for a company that did workshops all over the country, I jumped at it. I was living just two miles from Dallas-Fort Worth International Airport, and air travel was not nearly as laborious as it became later. I could do workshops or speeches on weekends or two day weekday trips and still have time to see all my clients. It was pretty much the perfect work for me at the time.

The trips kept me busy, but I needed that. It was a difficult time in my life. After talking with my husband, an engineer whom I had met in college, I had resigned my job at a rehabilitation hospital after 7½ years. Managed care had greatly reduced the number of patients for whom music therapy was covered by insurance, and I wanted to spend the next year writing some articles on my work. A month later, however, my husband announced that he wanted a divorce. Everything, it seemed for a while, was upside down. I was single and unemployed: two things I had never expected. I started therapy and soon learned I was clinically depressed, not as a response to the circumstances, but as an illness I had likely been struggling with since my teens. I had to face some tough truths and do some tough work. In a few months my husband was gone from our home, our two dogs had died (a sad coincidence), and I was still unemployed.

Fortunately, music therapists build wonderful communities. Two local therapists told me to apply for open part-time contracts at local facilities when they could have snapped them up themselves. One therapist who had been planning to squeeze an additional client into her load instead referred him to me. With this and other contracts I picked up, I was able to make it until the next fall, when a full-time school district job became available. I moved into an apartment, bought a cute little cockatiel ("Tony Vivaldi"), and started over.

So it was perfect timing that a publishing company contacted me and asked if I could join their team of speakers at conferences they hosted around the country. The company's founder was the father of a son on the autism spectrum and he had created the company to share information. Authors and others with experience in education and therapy formed a core group of speakers from which a community could choose, based on the topics they most wanted to hear about. He then organized a two-day conference in the community with a keynote speaker, four to five other presenters, and books for sale. When the original music therapy speaker was no longer available, I got the opportunity to join the group.

It was an enormous privilege. I traveled with them to cities from Portland, Maine to Honolulu, Hawaii. Each time, the group was slightly different, so I had the chance to hear many other speakers on a variety of topics such as communication tools, social stories, toilet training, sensory integration, and vocational support. The company founder always took the speakers out to a dinner between the two days of presentations and those conversations were usually fascinating. Some of my fellow speakers were autistic and they were typically blunt in describing both their own experiences and ways in which the rest of us could improve our work. It was refreshingly focused advice. I also met many parents, teachers and therapists in our audiences. As part of the contract with the speakers, the founder asked that we all be available in the breaks between any of the presentations over the two days, so that attendees could seek us out. The people I met gave me both new ideas (many parents, often out of desperation, write terrific songs) and challenging problems to investigate.

All of this traveling, meeting people who wanted to hear something new and helpful from me, was pretty gratifying at a time when my self-esteem had taken a big hit. It was good to be reminded that I had the ability to help others beyond my own clinical practice. The additional income didn't hurt either. But there were challenges to being seen as an expert, especially since I was sometimes the first music therapist the audience had ever met. One was to communicate the breadth of music therapy options for people on the autism spectrum. As I've mentioned in this book, there are at least three distinct approaches and many variations. Music therapists who work in the public schools usually structure sessions around composed and chosen songs that each address one or more goals. Other therapists use relatively unvarying rhythm-based protocols based on theories and research in neurological functioning. Still others build musical relationships through improvisation in a more long-term therapeutic process. And, of course, there are therapists like me who move between these approaches. As a speaker at these conferences, part of my assignment was to give the participants some concrete ideas they could implement in their homes, classrooms, and clinics. To do that, and to provide the research and theoretical justification that would convince the audience to give music and music therapy a try, I had to limit my focus. I chose to demonstrate and explain what I had found successful in a school setting: a song-based approach -- but I realized that I was leaving out some valuable and thought-provoking information.

***

Once my job in the school district started, I was able to bring the knowledge and ideas I'd acquired on the speaking circuit to my students and their teachers -- and to my own sessions. For example, after hearing a presentation by a vocational trainer, I realized that I had disregarded important aspects of how I presented material. The speaker had taught us to think about the difference between what we teach children with developmental disabilities and what they really need to know. When it takes you longer to learn any one thing, that thing had better be useful. Or, as he put it: "Why are you repeatedly asking your student what the cow says? Is he going to be a farmer?"

Considering this idea, I asked myself, "Why do my students need to know colors?" and instead of just colored dots or squares for a color song, I started using Jello boxes -- because one practical use of colors is to pick flavors. When my students were being asked to recognize and name coins, I remembered that the vocational instructor had told us that most of his clients didn't need to know the name of a coin -- just how to use it in a vending machine So I wrote a new song that paired each coin with the number of stars it would buy, focusing on relative value. For a goal about telling time, I wrote a clock song that traced the journey from home to school. Songs for practicing social conversation had only the most essential words that might actually occur in real life. And so on.

There's always so much more to learn.

***

It is fun to be in a profession in which you can have an almost immediate impact if you start sharing your ideas. On the other hand, putting your ideas out there for evaluation is scary. Furthermore, projects can get out of control in a hurry if you're not careful. Start with a few pet peeves, confront a few challenges, and suddenly you have a business partner, a small publishing enterprise, and you're being called to the stand to testify about music therapy in court!

As a music therapist in special education, I was writing a lot of songs. Many of the songs I found in books or heard people using weren't right for my students. The songs seemed to have been composed for the ear of the writer, not the children. For example, many were written and recorded for high soprano voices. But most children, even the most adorable, do not speak in a high range like that, and students with developmental disabilities often have lower voices than their neurotypical peers. When we sing outside our speaking range, we must engage several groups of muscles, in our diaphragm, larynx and mouth -- and that takes neurological planning that may not be present in people with cognitive and motor deficits. It didn't make sense to ask my students to try and produce words while also stretching their voice out of their usual range.

Another thing: the students I saw needed to hear things many times before absorbing them; many more repetitions over a longer period of time. Music provided a great medium for that kind of repetition and students often started to use words for the first time in songs. But many of the words in children's songs were set to melodies in a way that distorted them, especially when the words were "piggybacked" onto an old familiar melody. Try singing "My favorite color is red" to the first line of notes from *I've Been Working on the Railroad*. Some of the words will not sound like they do when they are spoken. A student of mine who learned words through a song like that might forever mispronounce them.

Sometimes the most important word was buried in the middle of a phrase, making it impossible to emphasize it without losing the pulse of the song. A word like that needed to be placed on a downbeat where it would receive a natural accent. Sometimes it was the music that made no sense. In one book, I found a song with the words "I'm walking up the stairs" -- to a melody of descending notes! If my students had no problems with speech or communication or cognition, these songs might have been fine, but my fellow school district therapists and I agreed: we had to do better.

So we wrote original songs, custom-designed for our students and their goals. We could test the songs on the spot and revise them if, for example, there wasn't enough time for a student to say a word, or when a harmonic progression could be tweaked to provide a better cue. Two of my colleagues, Kathleen Coleman and Debbie Dacus, put some of their songs together in a collection.

They printed it with a comb binding, gave it a bright pink cover and sold it at a regional conference. It was a hit.

About a year after "The Pink Book" made its debut, I was settling into my apartment, ready to start my new school district job. Kathleen came over one day with the gift of a drum she knew I could use as I started up my practice again. As we sat and talked, she proposed to me that she and I might publish a second songbook. At the time, she was just trying to find a project that would give me something new to focus on after the divorce and move. Her act of friendship had some unexpected consequences, however. As we developed the second songbook, we began to have other ideas as well. We should have expected this. Both of us were always full of advice and ideas, and once we started a discussion, it could go on for hours.

Within four years, we had produced an entire collection of materials: songbooks, visual aid kits, and instructional books for therapists and teachers. Each book came about organically; we simply transferred what we were doing in our work to print. For each song we shared the goals for which it had been written, but we encouraged users to be creative and change the songs to suit their students. We knew that every child is different and responds differently. Then we created a website and exhibited our books at conferences. Purely by addressing the needs of our own clients, we'd created a business. But while we were sometimes seen as experts, we were learning as much as we were sharing.

***

One of our projects had wider implications than we ever expected.

SEMTAP stands for Special Education Music Therapy Assessment Process. It is what's called an "eligibility" assessment: designed to help determine if students in special education should receive music therapy services. Kathleen and I developed and wrote it because we were hearing about, and getting involved in, increasingly contentious cases of parents fighting school districts. A child's response to music can often be profound and joyous, and many of the parents' arguments for music therapy to their child's IEP committees came off as emotional. On the other side, administrators did not view music therapy as a legitimate therapeutic profession like physical or occupational therapy, and they were dealing, as always, with finite budgets. These clashes sometimes went to a federally-mandated hearing called "due process" and sometimes beyond that to lawsuits. Tens of thousands of dollars were spent on lawyers and court fees that might have provided valuable therapy for a child. Some of those lawsuits did help the students, and a few ended up improving the circumstances for all children in special education. Many, however, resulted only in dollars lost.

Kathleen and I weren't trying to solve the entire problem when we got started. We simply wanted to find a way to answer questions from parents and administrators in North Texas where we worked. Kathleen, in particular, saw the value of a common strategy that all the local MT-BCs could use. We hunkered down, reviewed the special education disputes we and our colleagues had experienced, and tried to get to the essence of the conflict. We focused on the federal language regarding the provision of related services (music therapy being one of those) and built an assessment process that would answer the one question all the administrators had: How do I know that music therapy is required for this student to benefit from his or her special education plan? Using a model I had followed in assessing patients at the rehabilitation hospital, we developed a standardized process. Then we tried it out in several local districts and got feedback from all the parties. After a couple of years we made revisions and after sage advice from an editor, gave it an acronym. In 2002, we produced our *SEMTAP Handbook*.

We had no idea how it would be received. In fact, we kept going back to literature searches and email and phone inquiries, certain that someone had to have solved this problem before us. Our central idea -- to have the assessor test the same skills, in the same context, with and without music therapy -- was so simple that we were sure people had done it and couldn't believe it hadn't been formally proposed before. Even as we published the first copies of our *Handbook* and made our first presentations at conferences, we were sure we would be found out as copycats. We did end up with people who disagreed with our approach -- and we appreciated those disagreements -- but it turned out that our process was needed more than we ever imagined.

***

Once the SEMTAP was established and we were selling the handbook at regional and national conferences and through our website, Kathleen and I were called in to conduct the assessment in school districts where due process and lawsuits had been threatened. We discovered that some music therapists, with all good intentions, had encouraged parents to sue. They and the parents hoped to build the case for music therapy through the courts. Kathleen and I saw the SEMTAP as a change to avoid litigation. It did that (and continues to do so) in many, many cases. Our proudest moments were when the assessment yielded a "no" to music therapy and the parents said, "I'm not happy, but I understand" -- or when we recommended music therapy and an administrator said, "I finally understand why it is necessary to provide this service."

Fifteen years later, the SEMTAP has been used by hundreds of music therapists and school districts across the country. Kathleen and I are still astonished at how it all happened. It's wonderful to see that, even without a larger plan, we created something that has helped so many people. But it still makes me a bit anxious to be seen as an expert. After all, this is just one answer, not the only answer.

There's always so much more to learn.

There were times when a dispute had already reached due process before we were called. Kathleen dealt with dozens of these cases in Texas, and during the years that I traveled as a presenter and consultant, I was hired by out-of-town parents or school districts three times to conduct the SEMTAP: once in the Pacific Northwest, and twice in Midwest cities. The first two trips yielded positive results: the school district officials truly wanted to hear a logical rationale for the service and the local music therapists just needed to learn to use the assessment. In the last case, however, the situation was much more divisive, and would be familiar to many families who have fought for services in the public schools. After the district refused to conduct a music therapy assessment, the parents of a young female student with Down syndrome had the evaluation done by the student's private music therapist. The district refused to accept it, and the battle moved to due process.

In preparation for the hearing, the family attorney hired me to do a SEMTAP. Even though our process contained several steps that required time in the student's school, the district refused me access. I had to cobble together information from the files the parents had, and I had to do my "non-musical" observation at a private speech therapy session. The music therapy assessment was conducted in a hotel room. None of these were good conditions and I truthfully wrote in my report that the SEMTAP had not been accurately administered. I did observe the student's significant responses to music therapy and I reported that in detail. By the time I was done describing the student's status, the problems with the assessment in this case, and the student's specific behaviors with and without music, the report was 22 pages long.

A month later, the family brought me back to testify in their due process hearing. There was a three judge panel and testifying felt very much like being in a full-fledged trial. The family attorney's questions lasted about 30 minutes, but the school district attorney questioned me for 2 more hours. Following the advice Kathleen and I had written in the assessment handbook, I responded to all the questions by reading from my report, though I could tell this frustrated my questioner. Her queries were all designed to portray music therapy as a pseudo-therapy, justified only by positive feelings about favorite songs. Her problem was that the assessment findings were based on observed data and numerical results.

Finally, one of the judges interjected and asked, "Are you ever going to say anything that's not in those pages?" "No, sir," I said. "Well, then, you are excused," he declared, over the objections of the school attorney. Relieved, I exited. The eventual ruling was for the parents and their daughter, and the district was required to provide music therapy –- but it was sad to think that tens of thousands of dollars had been spent on that one decision.

More satisfying results came over the next few years, as the MT-BCs in that city school district began using the SEMTAP and, after a while, administrators began requesting its use. At a national conference held in that city two and a half years after my testimony, the district's special education administrator introduced Kathleen and me at our SEMTAP session. "We use the SEMTAP!" he declared proudly. We shook our heads in amazement.

***

After four years in the school district, I applied for and was offered a position as an assistant professor of music therapy at the university where I had received my master's degree and had been teaching as an adjunct. At the time there were no doctorates in music therapy, so a master's was considered the terminal degree. This meant I was awarded a tenure-track position like the professors around me. A year later, the other music therapy professor unexpectedly left to start a family and suddenly I was the head of our program, overseeing both undergraduate and graduate music therapy degrees. Having worked as an MT-BC for sixteen years at that point, I felt well-prepared to teach the clinical content of the courses. I was also a good writer, and could help my students write papers and theses. I was a "nationally-known" speaker and author of popular clinical materials. Perfect, right?

Well, the university staff from that time -- those whose job it was to process each student's grades, scholarship paperwork, internship contracts, etc. -- would tell you I was far from perfect. I had lots of clinical expertise, but almost no administrative experience. It was an incredible challenge for me to balance teaching and managerial tasks. A music therapy educator benefits from having a strong clinical background but when it comes down to it, a student needs someone who will lead them through not just the education, but also the bureaucracy of a college degree, in a timely and knowledgeable manner. I spent all four years at that university struggling to manage that aspect of the job.

For years I had resisted the idea of getting a doctorate. Many of the professors with doctorates I had met were those who had gone straight through school with perhaps five or six years of clinical experience, some as part of their education. As an experienced clinician, I was justifiably proud that I could teach my students what it was like to be "in the trenches." In a way, I thought the pursuit of a doctorate would negate the value of my experience. And I was in my forties and couldn't imagine going back to school.

My expertise and my perspective on teaching were hard-won. My own music therapy degree (a combination of certification requirements and masters-level work called a "masters-equivalency" program) had been supervised by a charismatic but volatile professor who had little to no clinical experience of his own. Music therapy programs were not yet regulated as stringently they are now by the American Music Therapy Association, and my fellow students and I were often thrown into clinical placements unsupervised. Our instrumental training consisted of one semester of piano from visiting faculty (my students now take at least 4 semesters each of piano and 2 semesters of guitar and hand percussion). Internships were not well-regulated either at that time, and for mine, I worked for 6 months at an inpatient psychiatric hospital where my supervisor was living with a former patient, in violation of numerous ethical codes. Much of my real music therapy education, therefore, had come after school, from generous and talented music therapy mentors in north Texas, and from my own independent study.

Fortunately, despite my stubbornness about a PhD, two professors that I admired from their work both as educators and clinicians urged me to enter the doctoral program at the University of Kansas. KU was, for many of us, the "mothership" of music therapy: its base in Lawrence, Kansas had been home to well-known writers and teachers in the field and our first organization, the National Association for Music Therapy. That connection put a crack in my resolve. Another dry, hot summer in north Texas made my native Great Lakes constitution weep, and anywhere north started to sound good. I realized that the doctorate would open up doors to teaching positions in places with all four seasons, and that after the divorce, I did not have to stay in Texas.

As I began to waver, I talked with my neighbor Velma, a retired special education teacher. After tea and Judge Judy (her favorite program) one afternoon, I told her about the offer from KU and my remaining question. "I can't imagine going back to school," I told her. "If I do this, I won't be done until I'm 48 years old!"

Velma smiled. "You'll be 48 years old anyway," she said.

I looked at her, puzzled.

"Do you want to wake up on your 48th birthday and be 'Dr. King,' or wake up and be in the same place you are today?" she asked.

I went home and filled out the KU application.

It was a good decision. I went into debt and I left many friends and familiar places behind, but the doctoral experience was extraordinary. I was able to focus on the neuroscience of speech and language, gain a deeper understanding of psychophysiology, study music philosophy, and improve my improvisation skills. I was able to research the impact of major and minor second dissonances on a listener's attention and measure the electrical activity (event response potentials: ERPs) in the brains of non-musicians as they listened to those same intervals. I gained a better understanding of many things I had seen in my clinical work and was able to develop new theories for my future practice and teaching.

I also observed the faculty at KU, especially my advisor, and worked on learning the administrative discipline and skills that had eluded me previously. Each of the professors in the KU music therapy program spent a full day each week outside the school in clinical work, and my admiration for that helped my stubborn heart open up to new ideas about how to be an academic leader. As a graduate assistant, I had a cadre of students to teach and supervise, so there were many opportunities to practice management skills. Organization was especially challenging in the tiny office I shared with another GA; it gave me an appreciation for the spacious professor's office I had left behind!

Today, back in a faculty position as an associate professor, I am better organized, but regularly aware of how little I know. Our field has exploded with theories, research, and interventions and I would love to be able to keep up. Music therapists draw not only from music therapy research but from studies in music cognition, music philosophy, music neuroscience, and music education. Each of us also follows non-music research that relates to our current clients, such as studies on autism, oncology, or pain management. We must continue to broaden our musicianship as well, so we can respond with ever more immediacy and creativity to our clients.

I also know I should contribute more. I know I need to write another article about the work I'm doing with speech-language therapists, but there are auditions to attend and committee work to complete. A colleague and I have successfully completed some projects focusing on elders with Alzheimer's, but there is more we want to do. Every day feels like a day that other music therapists are accomplishing more, publishing more, and learning more. In fact, I should stop writing this book immediately and start reading the two journals still in their mailing wrappers on my desk.

There is always so much more to learn -- and do!

CHAPTER SIX

Group Work

Group work is a common practice in therapy. Groups can enhance the therapeutic experience or provide more access to therapy when funds are limited. No matter what the rationale, music is an ideal medium for group therapy. A skilled therapist can engage people of varying ability levels in a single musical experience, strengthening each member's role in the group. The importance of each person's participation can keep group members connected to the present moment and to reality. The cooperation required to produce a single piece of music can create a unique bond between the participants, with the emotion of the music creating memories of support and success.

This chapter includes stories about several groups that I had the opportunity to lead over the years. They range from inmates at a county jail to families and patients in rehabilitation; from boys with autism, to elders with Alzheimer's and dementia. The common thread is music therapy interventions that are enhanced because participants are sharing the experience.

October
Lawrence, Kansas

I shook hands with the man leaving the music therapy group. "I can't tell you what this meant to me," he said. I looked and listened for hints of a con-artist, someone trying to play the game to get credit as cooperative, but found nothing. He seemed sincere. "You know what the most interesting part of the drumming was?" he asked, and then answered himself: "When we had to be quiet. It was hard but then the silence was kind of powerful. That was good."

While working on my PhD at the University of Kansas, I was thrilled to be able to start a music therapy pilot program at the country jail. Towns and cities that have university music therapy programs have an advantage over those that don't: the university's need for clinical training placements for their students. If there are not enough area music therapists who can act as supervisors for students, a university will send one of their graduate or doctoral students (who are already board-certified music therapists) to a facility to lead music therapy sessions. That MT-BC can then have students come, assist, and learn. Many university programs have a policy that restricts this "free" music therapy to a year or so. After that, facilities who want music therapy to continue are expected to hire an MT-BC.

A program coordinator at the jail, knowing about this routine, contacted the music therapy program at KU. The professor in charge of clinical education asked those of us who were doing supervision as part of paying for our graduate degrees if we were interested in conducting a pilot. A couple of us were, others were not. Not every therapist wants to do every type of work. For example, being part of a burn unit in a hospital where pain is a constant is draining. Providing hospice care means dealing with death and dying every day. In therapy with inmates, you face the conflict between working on rehabilitation and conveying positive messages and the reality of the often horrible crimes your clients have committed. Understandably, not everyone wants to do that.

The orientation my colleague and I went through at the jail was enlightening. I had previously visited a forensic psychiatric facility where a music therapist worked with prisoners who had mental illness or intellectual disabilities. That had been a rather whirlwind tour, however. This time the program director took the time to show us what the inmates were experiencing. We each spent some time inside a cell with a small window high in the wall, thin mattress on a concrete shelf, and complete lack of privacy for its toilet. We saw the exercise "yard," a fully enclosed concrete area on the second floor with netting overhead. There was a small learning annex for inmates who wanted to work on high school or college courses (this was a jail rather than a prison, so the longest length of stay was usually a year or two), and a library. Both those areas required multiple weeks of good behavior before admittance. The manager introduced us to the door locking system and showed us how to use our alarm buttons to call a guard from outside the room. We also learned that none of the inmates were allowed their own music: no boomboxes or personal audio devices. The only music they heard was that coming from whatever television show was playing in the common area.

My first group was comprised of 8 men from the maximum security unit who only knew that the session had something to do with music. I got the impression that they would have signed up for almost anything that got them off their unit for a while. Each had earned the privilege of attending the group, but I still was surprised by their calm and courteous demeanor. My student and I gathered them in a large circle and I gave a brief introduction, focusing on the fact that it was impossible to make a mistake in this group, and that all attempts would fit into our improvisations and songs. In a lot of group work, it is important to have the group agree upon rules. In this setting, most of the rules were already set by the jail itself, but I asked that they not express judgment about each other's music choices or preferences, and that they not criticize a person's attempts on the instruments or ideas about song lyrics.

My student helped me pass out drums and small percussion instruments, like cabasas, kokorikos, frame drums, and wood blocks. We also had three larger floor drums, the largest of which I would play to set the beat in deep bass tones. I had planned to lead a fairly free improvisation to start, with my steady rhythm providing structure and myself or my student using hand signals to get the group to play louder or more quietly, faster or slower, or to rest in silence for a beat or two. However, once I got the group going, one of the men asked a question, and immediately several more joined in.

"How do you know what to play on that drum?"
"Isn't there something called 4 time...or, wait a second, 4-4 time?"
"How do we stay together?"
"Do we all have to play at the same time?"

I was startled. I had assumed the men would relish the chance to play without specific boundaries or restrictions, but instead, they seemed to want to know more about the rules of music. Tentatively, I asked if they would like to know about rhythmic structure. A unanimous yes was the response.

We started with the idea of a 4-beat measure, chanting together, "1-2-3-4, 1-2-3-4..." and then tried it on the instruments. I shared with them that even college music majors begin to speed up unconsciously when they play a steady beat and that it helped to think of the subdivisions: "1 (and) 2 (and) 3 (and) 4 (and)..." We tried again and the beat stayed steady. Then I had them chant again, but leave the fourth beat silent. "1-2-3-[silence]-1-2-3-[silence]." We practiced not rushing into the second measure but instead letting the silence last a whole beat.

Once we had it while chanting, we tried it with the drums.

This success led to all sorts of combinations. Half the group would play the first four beats, the other half would respond. The whole group would play for 4 beats, be silent for 4 beats, and hope to play simultaneously when the third measure started. We played four measures at a time, leaving out the fourth beat in the first, the third beat in the second, and so on. My student took one of the floor drums and began beating more complex rhythms to liven up the music, as the rest of us worked to stay steady. And during all of this, each group member -- each inmate -- had to focus his attention, control any impulsivity, listen to others, and cooperate with the group to play in unison. Like the man who thanked me at the end of the group, they had to learn to appreciate the silences. These were exactly the skills that, according to the program director, the men needed to work on -- but we had been able to do that without being pedantic about it.

We ended the session with some blues songwriting. When we were finished, every member of the group came up to thank us individually. Gratitude, enjoyment, anticipation of the next group...every reaction was positive and more importantly, genuine. Of all the groups -- minimum and moderate security, women, the special population -- the men in the maximum security unit continued to be the most enthusiastic and eager to learn more.

June
Dallas, Texas

Ellie, the art therapist at our rehabilitation hospital, leaned over and spoke to the mother of one of our female patients. "Let's give her a chance to do it herself," she said, then added, "Could you help Brad over here? He needs someone to hold the paper while he draws on it."

Ellie and I were leading our Creative Arts Therapy evening group for patients and families and she was employing one of our favorite strategies: getting a parent to help someone other than their own child, reducing the hovering that was at once natural and problematic. The group had been a regular Tuesday night feature for 5 months now and we had discovered lots of ways for loved ones to share meaningful experiences with the patients without encouraging helplessness.

Eight patients and ten family members were seated around three tables in the large therapeutic recreation area in the basement of the hospital. We had opened with a song to a familiar tune that gave everyone a chance to fill in blanks with their names and feelings and connect as a group. Now we were in the first half of the session, working with art materials. Each patient was using both sides of a paper plate to make two faces: a face for the way they saw themselves, and a face for how they thought others saw them. Some of the patients had spinal cord injuries or amputations; they were immediately able to understand the concept but needed help with using adapted tools to complete their faces. Other patients had brain injuries and needed explanations or reminders of the goal of the project. Some patients needed help with everything. We had various ways to describe the task, various definitions of success, and any effort was a positive one.

As each patient finished his or her "face plate," Ellie and I circulated, learning what the faces were meant to convey. Sitting down with Bob, one of my music therapy patients, I listened to his halting explanation. His brain injury had resulted in both aphasia (disruption in the use of language) and apraxia (affecting his speech), but because the neural pathways for singing familiar songs were distinct from those, he was able to sing more intelligibly than he spoke. On his plate that evening, he had drawn one face with a scribbled, mangled mouth -- how others saw him --- and on the other side, a face on which the mouth was replaced with a crude drawing of a guitar. He smiled at me and we sang together a fragment of a song from that afternoon's music therapy session, sharing the understanding that music was providing him an outlet and a rare feeling of normalcy.

During the second half of the group, I helped everyone create a song in which the patients could show and share their art and everyone could encourage one another. The songwriting process was not about an end product -- though we did sing together by the end -- but rather a safe place to discuss the meaning behind the faces everyone had drawn. The rhythm and harmony of the music helped each person stay focused on the task. Before the session I had collected groups of instruments with contrasting sounds (bells and drums) imagining that perhaps we would use distinct sounds to accompany the two sides of the plates. By the time we had all experimented with song ideas, however, the different accompaniments were used to compliment first a patient's statement about his or her face, and then the family member's response.

"Everybody sees I can't talk."
"I still love you and want to know how you feel."

"I am happy but my face is sad."
"I'm glad you told me!"

After the group ended, Ellie and I sat down to document the session together. Although healthcare paperwork can sometimes be tedious, or difficult to complete as quickly as needed, this documentation work never failed to inspire us. We had designed a unique reporting format which allowed us to not only chart appropriately in the medical record, but also to answer questions particular to creative arts therapies. We had begun to see some patients progress in ways we hadn't expected and which would never have been noted in our standard paperwork. The ideas and discussion this process provoked usually kept us sitting at one of the tables late into the evening. Eventually our collaboration led to an article published in one of the music therapy journals.

On that evening, we were focused on three of the scales we had developed, because half of the clients had made leaps in progress in those areas during the session. Bob had clearly "expressed personal issues" with his face drawings, and for the first time, he had done it with no assistance or prompting from anyone. He had moved from a "4" to a "1" on that scale in the past two weeks, from requiring assistance in creating a product at all, to independently communicating something important through a visual metaphor. Meanwhile, Sheri's mom, Sue, who had been unable or unwilling to let Sheri try anything herself the previous week, had spent the entire session helping Jamal who then made gains in independence because of Sue's assistance. And Rory had, for the first time, recognized the drawing he'd been helped to make as representing him. The injury to the frontal and parietal lobes of his brain had disconnected him from being aware of himself and his actions, so this was a significant development.

It was exciting to see that this progress and improvements in most of the patients and their families took place in an atmosphere that the participants viewed as a friendly, relaxed social time, not therapy. After a full day of formal therapy, no one wanted to fill their evening with more hard work. Yet through the joy of creating and the freedom of choices that art and music provided, each person was continuing to move towards recovery.

February
Dallas, Texas

Five boys on the autism spectrum, each with additional cognitive challenges, were my first group of the day. Their classroom was half of a portable building on an urban school district's elementary school campus. The boys were 7 and 8 years old and in a program that helped them learn to organize themselves through the use of black-and-white picture symbols. Each day when they came in from the bus, they were handed cards with a picture of their locker. They went to their locker, put their coats away, put the "locker" card in an envelope and took the card attached to the front of that envelope. This second card's picture directed them to one of the work stations in the classroom where each would have individualized schoolwork to complete. On Tuesdays they worked on that until they came to music therapy.

All five boys had trouble expressing themselves verbally, though they didn't have aphasia or apraxia. Most of what they said was an echo of another person's speech. They also were anxious about change and did not cope well when they felt strong emotions, dissolving into crying tantrums or being so excited that they ran around the room knocking things over. In music therapy, however, there were fewer behavioral problems, probably because the music drew them into a common experience and the familiar, predictable structure let them feel in control.

When working with a group of younger children, especially any that have attention or behavioral challenges, I like to use the music to keep everyone involved, even if it's important to work with each student individually. Music provides several forms that work well for this. In a verse and chorus format, I can use a short verse to work with one student, then have everyone sing and/or play for the chorus. Next verse, next student, then everyone back in for the chorus. I can use a rondo format (A-B-A-C-A-D-A...), where the "A" part is for the whole group and can be something as simple as "Hey Hey Hey!" Using this, I can do something distinct with each student (B, C, and D), even something in which the music is different, because everyone comes together on the A part which stays consistent.

The session I did with this group of boys had two regular songs that were structured like that: one for "hello." and one for "how are you?" The songs provided a safe place to practice some pretty confusing things: social conversation and rules of sharing and taking turns. Many students on the autism spectrum learn quickly but very specifically: they don't generalize one situation to another. So when their teacher greets a student every day with "Hi, Matthew!" he knows to respond with "Hi Mrs. Thomas," but when another teacher in the hall greets him, she says "Matthew! How's it going?" -- and that seems like a completely different situation. When the responses are that complicated for Matthew, he's going to be unlikely to initiate the conversation himself.

Our greeting song began with my singing something like:

Hello! I'd like to sing with you –
I'd like to shake your hand.
My name is Betsey,
And your name is.....

at which point the student could say his name and shake my hand. If touching was difficult for a student, as it could be for those with sensory integration challenges, I could change the words to "Let's wave our hands for 'hi!' – and, in fact, I often changed the words. By doing that, I was demonstrating that greetings could have many forms. The underlying music, however, stayed consistent: same melody, same chords, same rhythm for the accompaniment. The music became the "category" students could recognize even while the specifics changed.

When we moved on to the "how are you?" portion of our opening, I was able to use music to distinguish emotions. The song started: "How are you, [name], how are you?" The student I named picked a picture card (like the ones they used for tasks in the classroom) that had a face with an emotion. I played the next part of the song reflecting that feeling. If a student picked "excited," I played fast and lively. If a student picked "sad," I changed the accompaniment to a minor key and slowed down. Tired was very slow, with pauses for yawning. Angry was also in a minor key, but with loud aggressive strums on my guitar. The student would say the emotion word out loud and then the rest of us would respond, singing in the style I was playing: "Tim... is feeling... tired ...today."

At the beginning of the semester, the boys seemed to pick the cards at random. After a few weeks, I could tell that some of them were associating the feeling with the style of music, because they would pick a card and then change their posture or expression to prepare themselves for the way I was about to play and sing. They weren't yet picking a feeling card based on their own emotion at the time, but they understood that each face represented a different feeling. Music was an effective and efficient way of communicating this distinction.

We continued to sing these songs throughout the year, even when other aspects of the session changed according to the individual academic goals the students had. The classroom teacher used fragments of the songs during the week to remind the students that they were in a greeting situation, or to encourage them to express an emotion. After all, doing these things in the music therapy session was fine, but if they couldn't carry the concepts into the rest of their day, I wasn't doing them much good.

One day, early in the second semester, I found out that at least one of our students was "generalizing:" taking the skills out of the session and into his life. I arrived a little early to the portable classroom and was already there when Tim's mother dropped him off. I introduced myself and she said, "Oh! You must be singing about feelings!" I asked how she knew that, and she told me that two evenings earlier, Tim had asked to watch a videotape right before they were going to sit down to dinner. She had told him there wasn't enough time. Apparently his usual reaction to such a refusal was to melt down into a tantrum. On that night, however, he stood in the center of the room, and stomped his foot on the floor as he sang "I. Am. ANGRY. I am ANGRY!" She said she'd never been so thrilled to have one of her children "talk back" to her.

A few weeks later, I heard another story. I was setting up a music therapy session in another classroom in the district. The aide in that classroom asked me about one of the boys who was working on greetings in the early session. "Do you do music therapy with Harrison?" I said that I did. She told me, "I drive his bus in the afternoon. You won't believe what he did the other day. He came up the steps of the bus and stopped right next to me and started singing.

"Hello, I'd like to sing with you --
I'd like to shake your hand.
My name is Harrison,
and your name is – "

She continued. "So I knew the song from hearing you sing it, but I was so surprised --especially because he sang his own name, when he's only ever heard your name in the words. It took me a second, but I said, 'Janelle.' And you know what he did? He sang, 'How are you, Janelle? How are you?'"

We both threw our arms up in the air in excitement.

"Did you tell him how you were?" I asked.

"Yeah, but he had already gone back to his seat."

We laughed. Harrison didn't have all the pieces of the social routine down, but he had taken a big step.

March
Rochester, New York

Paula shifted in her seat, looking back towards the exit to the room. "I…is there?….I need a ride home, so…." She began looking around her chair. "Where is my purse? I have to have an apple or I'll starve…" Her voice began to crack with worry.

I inwardly scolded myself. During this opening period in our session for a small group of patients with dementia and Alzheimer's, it was important to move smoothly from one song to another. Any significant pauses between them -- and I had just created one by taking the time to shift my chair -- gave Paula's anxiety a chance to assert itself.

I quickly played an opening chord and began singing, "God bless America…" My graduate assistant, Terri, and the other two clients, Tom and Lorene, joined in. Paula's attention shifted immediately and she began singing in a clear soprano, smiling and swaying with the music. There was no sign of any of her previous concerns. The group continued singing the song and as I added rhythm to my accompaniment suggesting military drums, I saw Tom and Paula's posture straighten.

This group of clients was part of a pilot program that my colleague, Laurie, and I were running out of the music therapy clinic at our college. A donor had provided us with funds to do some work outside of our regular teaching and clinic responsibilities. We were seeking to collect data and evidence that would support the use of true music therapy in our area's long-term care facilities. We knew that the few music therapists employed in nursing homes and the like were too often used as entertainers or for recreational music, with groups much too large to address individual goals. Yet we also knew that a growing body of research demonstrated small group and individual music therapy could have significant and sustained effects on the cognitive, emotional, and physical status of people with Alzheimer's and dementia.

Today, Laurie was out sick, and our graduate assistant was responsible for collecting data, so I was leading the session on my own. This was not a big problem; most music therapists work on their own and can do effective, targeted work with a larger group than three people. We had, however, planned some of our strategies with both of us involved: one person on accompaniment and one person directly interacting with the clients. When possible, this can be a richer experience for the clients. The first strategy following the openings songs was one of these. We put floor drums -- large djembes or dumbeks -- in front of each client. Laurie played and sang a bebop tune at the piano as I cued each client to take turns "soloing" (beating the drum) in the natural pauses in the song. I had been gradually decreasing my cues over the past couple of weeks as our clients became more independent in listening for their opening and playing when it was time.

That was the wonderful thing we were seeing in this group. We had expected, based on the research, to see less anxiety, more physical involvement, and probably more talking or other vocalizations from our clients. What we hadn't anticipated was the amount of new learning that these, and other clients in the program, were demonstrating. During 6 months of once-a-week music therapy sessions, we were seeing each client -- despite his or her degenerative disease -- learn parts of the session routine. They were recognizing each other, though they only saw each other once a week. They could not tell us what was coming or what was required in a particular intervention, but showed increasing independence in carrying out their tasks. They were gaining new procedural memories.

Terri helped me place the drums in front of each client. Tom, a former music educator, immediately reached out with both hands, and thumped his djembe. Lorene had her own technique: she reached out and tapped the tips of her fingers on the drumhead. Paula, however, looked at the drum and us, confused. "I don't know how to play this," she said. Terri reached over and tapped the head of the drum then gestured for Paula to put her hands there. Then she took her place in front of them with her own drum, and I went to the piano. Now another challenge presented itself.

I am not a good pianist. My music therapy education, which occurred before academic programs were as closely overseen by our association as they are now, did not place an emphasis on piano. As a string player, guitar came much more easily to me and no one required me to gain an equal facility on piano. Today, my own students will learn both instruments, as well as some percussion skills and will be able to implement more aspects of music therapy because of it.

As for me, I've improved on my own over the years, but I'm not as facile as Laurie and I can't interact as smoothly with a group when I'm playing the keyboard. So as I stood at our electronic piano that day, I was more focused at first on my hands and fingers than on our clients. I got the song started and played up to the first pause. Terri cued Lorene to play, but tentatively. This was her first time as a leader in this group. Now I had two things on my mind other than the clients: my piano playing and my suggestions for Terri. It was no surprise that my next notes were mangled and I struggled to find the rhythm. This was not music that was going to inspire or cue anyone. After one more attempt, I knew I had to put the focus back where it belonged.

"You know what?" I said to the clients. "I'm terrible at this!" They laughed along with me. "Let me get my guitar, " I continued, "and we'll start again." Terri looked relieved as I came and sat down. I looked around and had an idea. "Let's put all the drums together and gather around."

Terri helped me put all the drums together in a tight grouping and help the clients move up and around them, each still in front of a single drum, but close to the others. I began the song accompaniment again, but didn't even get through the first phrase before the clients began playing their drums. I had changed the setup, so none of them were following the previous plan. As I considered stopping and resetting, Tom suddenly reached out and whacked Lorene's drum with his right hand, grinning mischievously. She was startled, but quickly -- with a playful look on her face -- reached over and whacked his drum right back! I kept the song going, using a nod of my head to ask Terri to help keep Paula playing. Before she could do that, Tom reached over to Paula's drum and gave it a whack. Paula looked at me and I smiled, nodding back at Tom and his drum as I sang. It took her a moment, but she reached over and hit Tom's drum, and soon all three clients were beating their own drums and, occasionally, each other's. Lorene and Tom were smiling and Paula, though she still seemed a bit confused, was participating in the game. Best of all, they were looking at each other, leading the music. Terri and I were in the background.

The following week, Laurie and I kept this part of the session intact and while Tom again took the lead in sharing drums, everyone participated right away. Paula even began to smile and scrunch her shoulders when she "snuck" a beat onto Tom's drum. Tom would respond with encouragement: "Ah! You got me!" and play hers in return. This was one of the times Lorene stood up and, stepping into the open area behind her chair, began to dance. As Laurie and I kept the music going, Tom stood up and joined her, soon coming back for Paula. With Terri's encouragement and physical support, Paula joined them and they danced in a circle together.

CHAPTER SEVEN

Keeping the Beat

Music and neurological research over the last fifteen years has confirmed what musicians, music therapists, and others have observed for much longer: that a strong rhythmic beat primes and facilitates movement. We now know that our responses to a steady pulse occur at a preconscious level. In other words, our movement doesn't initially improve because we like the rhythm or the music, but because structures and networks in our brains synchronize with the beat.

A little over ten years ago, music therapy strategies based on such neurological information were codified in an approach called Neurologic Music Therapy. The researchers who established NMT, led by Dr. Michael Thaut, made the important connections between experiences like the ones I describe in this chapter and the neuromotor operations of the brain. They developed a labeling system for strategies based on the goals of the patient, worked with neurologists to further explore the neural roots of musical responses, and began a 4-day training institute. The neurological research has been groundbreaking in our field, and the training has helped many music therapists view their work differently.

Some music therapists use NMT as their primary orientation and insist that NMT is unique in its approach and research base, but there are music therapists all over the world who study neuroscience and develop strategies and protocols based on research. And, as you can see in the stories below, most of which happened before NMT was developed, music therapy clients have been showing their therapists the power of the beat for a long, long time.

September
Rochester, New York

Ann and I walked up the sidewalk to the front door of the one-story brick house on the west side of town. I was tagging along to observe Ann do a home-care physical therapy session with one of her clients. We were curious as to how music therapy might be incorporated into some of these sessions to improve the client's motivation and possibly his physical abilities.

Mr. M greeted us at the door. He had Parkinson's disease but was still walking ("ambulatory") and living with his wife independently. His home care visits were designed to help him maintain that status. Ann came to the house twice a week and led Mr. M through stretching and mobility exercises. On her previous visit she had obtained his permission for my observation. "Call me Ed," he said.

I really was intending only to observe. I hoped to gather enough information about how a home care PT session was conducted to create some sample music therapy interventions that we could try at a later date. The only problem with this plan was that when I get in a room with a client, it's almost impossible for me not to offer something musical, even if I don't have my guitar or any of my other usual music therapy tools.

***

The impetus for my curiosity about collaborating with PT in home care came from previous experience. One such memory: I was sitting at one of the tables in the large therapeutic recreation space of the rehab hospital, having just returned from the medical center across the street. The group I'd led on the bone marrow transplant unit had gone particularly well and the unit administrator had just told me that she'd received approval to continue the group for another 6 months.

I was on a high after that and ready to tackle anything -- and anything came through the door from the PT area. A frail elderly man with a small beard and mustache that made him look a little like a pictures of a Civil War veteran was being helped into the room by two therapists on either side of him. It was obvious that although his legs could bear his weight, he had a motor impairment that was preventing him from moving them to walk. Each therapist was helping to hold him up: Kim, the physical therapist, was nudging each foot forward with her foot behind his heel, and Erica, a neuropsychologist, was trying out various verbal cues.

The research on rhythm and gait (walking) was in its earliest stages, but I, like most music therapists, had seen the evidence in clients in our own sessions. I walked over to the trio coming through the door and asked, "May I try something?" Kim looked over at Erica and then nodded.

"Hi, Mr. Jordan?" I said, reading his hospital bracelet. He looked up at me. "My name is Betsey. Follow me!"

Immediately I began singing and marching backwards, exaggerating my movement so my feet were stomping the floor and emphasizing the words that fell on the beat.

Mine *eyes* have *seen* the *glo*ry
of the *com*ing *of* the *Lord*
He is *tramp*ling *out* the *vin*tage
where the *grapes* of *wrath* are *stor*ed.

Within the first line, Mr. Jordan had straightened up. By the second line, he was marching towards me, his steps smaller and lighter, but independent. Kim and Erica kept a hold of him for balance, but Mr. Jordan walked on his own.

He hath *loos*ed the *fate*ful *light*ning

of his *terri*ble swift *sword,*
His *truth* is *march*ing *on*....

I had walked backwards in a curve so as to avoid the recreation tables and had led the trio to double doors that led out into the hospital hallway. I backed off and they continued down the hallway, singing on their own.

Glory! Glory! Hallelujah!
Glory! Glory! Hallelujah!
Glory! Glory! Hallelujah!
His truth is marching on...

***

Back at the home PT session, I followed Ed and Ann into one of the home's bedrooms where he sat down on the edge of the bed and she knelt beside him. I found a chair a few feet away and watched as she began helping him with a series of stretches. After some which were done seated, Ed lay back on the bed and Ann began working on stretches that involved his hip flexors. Ed had seemed uncomfortable during the early stretches but now he was wincing. I saw him look at me and couldn't help asking, "Would you like a song to see it will help you relax?"

"That would be great," he said, and we discussed options before settling on hymns.

I began singing *His Eye is on the Sparrow*, watching the rhythm Ann established with the stretches and finding a way to link up the 3/4 time of the song with Ed's leg movements. Ed joined me in the chorus and the act of singing deepened his breathing. We sang another verse and chorus and then paused.

"Your legs were more relaxed just now," Ann said to Ed. "The singing really does help," Ed replied. We agreed on another hymn and used it to accompany the rest of his stretching exercises.

From there we moved into the dining room where Ann worked on some sitting and standing with Ed while I observed. With those exercises done, Ann led Ed into the kitchen. Ed knew the routine and positioned himself facing the counter with his palms flat on the edge. Ann took a large coffee can from the cabinet and put it on its side, on the floor, just to the right of Ed's right leg.

"You know what to do," she told Ed, and he lifted his right leg so that his foot was higher than the can, then pushed his foot over it and down so he was now standing with it between his feet. He had a difficult time lifting his leg and there was a noticeable tremor as he extended it to the other side of the coffee can. Once he was "astride" it and Ann instructed him to lift the leg up and over and back to its original position, he again had trouble starting the movement and controlling it. Each repetition of this exercise took a different amount of time as Ed tried to control and smooth out the movement of his leg.

Watching this, I tried an approach that has been codified by NMT as "patterned sensory enhancement (PSE)." Using my voice (and really wishing I'd brought my guitar), I sang a strong note to start ("boom!"), then made a siren of my voice, going first up and then down in an arc that mirrored the arc Ed wanted to take with his foot over the coffee canister. I ended my siren on another strong note as Ed's foot came to rest on the other side. As I kept up this pattern, matched to the general speed of Ed's efforts, his leg became steadier and the movement smoother and more efficient. The effect was almost instantaneous and the three of us smiled at his success.

***

Dallas. The home of my first private client. Brian was 14 and a survivor of a severe brain injury. He used a wheelchair and required some support from a padded head rest to keep his head level and steady. We were in the middle of our session and I was working with him on a goal set by his physical and occupational therapists: to move his left hand across his body and back again. This action is called "crossing the midline" and is difficult for some people with brain injuries because it requires shifts in control and perception between the brain's two hemispheres.

During the week prior to the session, I had been struggling with how to address this objective. Brian couldn't speak, but his facial expressions indicated that all activities around this goal were his least favorite. I had tried using his favorite country songs as a background but he hadn't responded. He liked using his left arm for musical tasks like strumming an autoharp or playing a drum -- as long as the arm stayed on the left side of his body. So what, I asked myself, might help him get that arm across the midline?

The idea came at a stop light and I drove from one client's house to another. Just as I hit the brakes, the rock station I was listening to cued up Billy Squier's *Everybody Wants You*. It had come out 3 years earlier and the opening had an instant effect on many in my generation: the driving guitar and drums made it impossible to sit still. Whether it was your head or your hands or your legs: something was nodding, tapping, stomping. I realized that what I needed for Brian were not necessarily *his* favorite songs (external motivation), but songs that had a rhythm that would hopefully compel him to move the arm (internal propulsion).

At our next session I cued up the song and used words and gestures to encourage Brian to follow my hand. At first I stayed on his left, simply moving slightly side to side every two beats ("half-time."). Then I placed his hand on top of mine and continued the small movement. As we continued I expanded the distance we traveled, my hand providing the initial lift and movement, but Brian moving too, so his hand didn't fall off mine. As the music with its strong rock beat continued, Brian's movement with mine became more confident and I was able to further widen the distance between the two points on the table, eventually crossing the midline. By the time the song was over, my hands were in my lap and Brian was moving his hand back and forth on his own.

***

Ed's session was almost over, but Ann had one more assessment to do -- and an idea. The assessment was called a "TUG test" for "Timed Up and Go." It would assess Ed's balance and mobility and Ed knew its procedure well. First, he sat down in a chair. When Ann said "go" and started a stopwatch, Ed stood up, walked to a spot she had marked 10 feet away, turned around, walked back, turned again, and sat down. Ann clicked the stopwatch off. "24 seconds," she announced. "Now, let's try it again with some music."

Once again wishing I had brought some instruments with me, I decided to use my voice and clap to emphasize the beat. Ed had been in the Air Force, so my mind went immediately to its theme song ("Off we go...into the wild blue yonder..."). "When you hear the music start," I said to Ed, "go"- - and I launched into a vocal fanfare like the trumpets would play before the song. The instant the fanfare started, Ed stood up and as the song began, he marched forward to the mark, turned, and returned to his chair. Ann clicked her stopwatch off again. "17 seconds!" she exclaimed.

Count off 7 seconds to yourself and you'll see how significant a difference music with a strong beat made for Ed. Try it yourself the next time you have a physical task to complete. Music is more than an accompaniment; it facilitates movement. We now have the neurological explanation, but for people whose movement has been compromised, the impact of music can seem like a miracle.

INTERLUDE

Perception

Thirty years. Practicing music therapy and being in musical relationships with my patients and clients has always been a joy. It's frustrating, though, that I still run into many of the same questions and misunderstandings about the profession that I did when I started. At this point, I have answers ready for the most common queries and misstatements, but sometimes I wish I didn't have so much experience!

"Are you the Music Lady?"

This is a question I've heard often throughout my career. It's usually posed by someone who sees me in a hallway or an elevator, guitar slung across my back, instruments in a bag at my side. The question isn't meant to be insulting. It's usually asked with an air of positive expectation. People like music and they are happy to see it come to a hospital or a nursing home or a school.

When I hear this question I always hope I will have one minute with the person who is asking. In that one minute, I can give her a brief explanation of what I actually do and raise awareness for my small but important profession. Every little bit counts.

"I'm the music therapist here. You're right, there are volunteers who come in to lead sing-a-longs or play on the unit. That's so great for the patients. But I'm part of the medical team. I'm here to work with the patients who have a particular problem that can be addressed through music, like recovering speech after a stroke, or managing pain, or coping with being in the hospital."

***

"Oh, we already have music therapy here at the Medical Center. We have a guitarist who plays in the lobby and sometimes at the bedsides of the patients. It's really beautiful."

"Oh, we already have music therapy here at Golden Manor! We have iPods with personal playlists for many of our elders. They love it!"

"Oh, we already have music therapy for our veterans' group. We have a songwriter who comes in and helps the vets write songs. They get a lot out of it."

As a music therapist, I'm thrilled that each of these places knows that music is beneficial and therapeutic. I'm sure that each of these programs is valuable and I hope they will continue. I'm well aware, however, that none of them are actually providing music therapy. If I were able to work in any of those situations, I'd want those same musical offerings to continue – in *addition* to music therapy. The problem is that many people don't know the difference between the ways music can be part of health and education.

Many people use music in their own lives therapeutically. Others share music and bring joy to people in difficult circumstances. These folks don't need someone trained in assessment, in developing music and music strategies to match a person's goals, in how to work as part of a health care team.

But some people, at certain points in their lives, *do* need that. Some children on the autism spectrum respond most strongly to music that is composed for and improvised with them. Some adults, trapped by addiction, can access their feelings only through meaningful songs and need someone who can use that to promote recovery. Some elders who are agitated and combative due to dementia can be calmed only through musical communication that adjusts to them, moment to moment. Sometimes music therapy, provided by an MT-BC with professional training and resources, is the best way to reach and help people.

Think about this: Depending on one's cognitive status and stress level, music can start out as soothing or energizing but become overstimulating after a period of time, causing anxiety or distress. Simply lowering the volume or turning off the music can help, but sometimes it's more important for the tempo to slow down, or for the accompaniment to become simpler. That can't happen with recorded music or with live music played by someone who can't recognize the signs of overstimulation. If the Medical Center or Golden Manor had a music therapist, the MT-BC would be constantly checking for nonverbal reactions and would be experienced in adjusting live music. While some patients would benefit most from a personal playlist, and others would enjoy volunteer musicians, an MT-BC could work with those who required special attention and responsiveness.

For example, some patients need to be more alert, or more social, or increase physical activity -- and research shows that active music making is more effective than passive. Some of those patients are able to participate independently in a music group, like a rock band or bell choir, and some initiate their own participation during a performance by clapping hands, singing along, or dancing. People with greater physical or mental impairments, however, often need different kinds of assistance. The music therapist at a place like Golden Manor would know how to take the simplest musical offerings from those residents (one spoken word, one beat on a drum), build reinforcing musical experiences around them, and gradually help them increase their contributions to the music. The MT-BC could help those residents with more challenging goals and improve their health status, emotional state, and quality of life.

Songwriting is a great outlet, and a gifted songwriter can be a great resource. But there will always be people who aren't ready to put their feelings into words. They may be able to express themselves more fully in an instrumental improvisation. And there are people for whom songwriting will unlock memories and emotions, some stressful or negative. That person needs the safety of a professional who knows how to respond and when to refer to another professional with specialized skills.

"I'm so glad your facility recognizes how much music can add to a healthcare environment. Let me tell you about how a music therapist can *add* to your programming, especially in working with people with more significant challenges."

***

"Music therapy is like a bubble bath. It feels good, but so what?"

"Music therapy isn't supported by enough randomized control studies. How can I recommend it?"

The research we use in music therapy work comes from several fields of study: among them, music cognition, music education, music neuroscience and music therapy itself. Our decisions are based on more than published research, however. Like any therapy that considers itself evidence-based, we also rely on our observations and on the client's perspective and desires. And, as musicians, we also listen and respond musically, and notice our client's musical behavior and creativity. We document our sessions carefully and make plans based on all these factors.

So yes, music therapy usually feels good, but its impact is much broader than that because it is based on careful design, and because MT-BCs know how to focus on more than one area of need. Music therapy *has* been shown to be effective in randomized control trials (often considered the gold standard for experimental research) as well as other kinds of quantitative studies, and it has a rich cache of qualitative studies as well that often describe what we do much better than a carefully controlled experiment. And while the field does not have as large a body of research as some other allied health professions, it is comprised of a smaller number of professionals, most of them working full-time as clinicians. Considering this, there is an impressive amount of research demonstrating how effective music therapy is in areas like neonatal intensive care, children's oncology, special education and elder care.

"Music therapy is supported by both quantitative and qualitative research as well as professional documentation -- and its uses of music are supported by research in music cognition, music neuroscience, and many allied health professions. Can I send you some links?"

***

"The school district isn't going to provide music therapy for this student. You didn't give a standardized test and we only accept standardized tests."

As the author of an assessment tool, I have heard this statement directly and been told about it by hundreds of parents, teachers, and other music therapists. It's not a legally correct statement (according to federal law), but it is somewhat understandable. We've all been conditioned to expect that evaluations will result in numbers, in a score. We expect to be compared to a large group and ranked according to our performance or status. In testing, this is called a norm-referenced assessment. What makes music therapy amazing, however, is also what makes it impossible to measure in that way.

Standardized tests measure one thing: your vocabulary, the range of motion in your right arm, the number of minutes it takes for you to put a puzzle together. A physical therapy test measures physical ability. A speech-language assessment measures communication skills.
A music therapy evaluation, however, does not measure musical skills. Musical skills aren't necessary for a person to benefit from music therapy. A music therapy assessment is specific to what you need, today, and its purpose is to find out if music therapy will help you get you there. And when you are in a music therapy session, the interventions won't just be affecting one aspect of your life (one "domain" as the professionals call it). Music that supports a physical task can also make you more alert. Music that helps with a speech challenge can

also give you an emotional lift. A music therapy eligibility assessment results in data ("the student performed the skill 25% of the time without music and 40% of the time with music"), but it doesn't give scores that can be compared to hundreds or thousands of other students. It measures how well music therapy helps one particular student achieve his or her particular goals. This is what's called a criterion-referenced assessment.

"Mr. Thomas, if I gave this student a standardized test for musical skills, it would not give you the information you want. You don't want to know if Jeremy can keep a steady beat. You want to know if music therapy is necessary for Jeremy to progress in his individualized education plan. To do that, I have to evaluate how well music therapy works on the specific objectives you've set for him."

***

Oh, you're a music therapist? Isn't that where you play Mozart and people get smarter?

Over the years, I've heard and seen many gimmicks and programs that purport to use music for some startling results. Some take a single research result and magnify it out of proportion, frustrating the researchers and fooling the public. Some take traditional healing practices out of their cultural context and package them as quick fixes. What usually distinguishes them is their "one size fits all" approach. It's an enticing claim: listen to this specially engineered recording (for example) and you will sleep better/learn a foreign language/lower your blood pressure/get smarter. But "one size fits all" does not work with music. Each person has genetic, cultural, societal and personal reasons for preferring one piece of music over another.

In most people's lives, there is a song, or even an entire genre, that they don't like, despite the fact that it is popular and a favorite of many of their friends. For me, Pachelbel's Canon in D is one of those pieces. It's beautiful, but its popularity means that, when I was playing violin I was called upon to play it all the time. I'm tired of it to the point of annoyance. And then there's 1980's music. I was in my 20's during that decade, and research tells us that music from our 20's is often our preferred music throughout our adult lives. I do like lots of '80's music, but if I hear *Lady in Red* or the Human League's *Don't You Want Me?* I actually feel a bit ill. Something in the timbres and harmonies doesn't sit well with me. I don't know why, but I hope no one ever puts them on a playlist for me, assuming I'll respond positively just because they were hits in the 1980's.

Our music preferences and reactions have many sources unique to each individual. Music research has shown us that we ascribe more emotions to music that has unexpected elements and that we prefer music more as those unexpected moments increase -- that is, until the point at which too much uncertainty leads to a dramatic *drop* in preference. But "unexpected" means something different for every listener. Someone who has grown up listening to basic popular music will prefer certain pop songs due to harmonic or melodic or rhythmic surprises, but they likely will find jazz too chaotic. On the other hand, I grew up with jazz, and I played quite a bit of modern atonal music at my conservatory. So for me, many pop songs are *too* predictable to get an emotional response out of me unless they are linked to a particular memory. The fact is, no one can predict a musical effect without knowing the person for whom it is intended.

Music therapy would probably be much more well-known if it consisted of packaged programs that were guaranteed to produce certain results. Instead, it is an approach that is based on personal relationships and personalized therapy. We work one person at a time, one moment at a time. It's more difficult to explain, but infinitely more rewarding.

"The Mozart Effect? That's something that was popular but not supported by evidence. Music therapy is really different. Each case is different and fascinating. Can I give you an example?"

CHAPTER EIGHT

The Music of Speech and Language

Speech and language recovery is the area of work about which I am most passionate these days, and my endless fascination often means that I will talk with almost anyone about the latest neuroscience research, or a new music therapy technique I've been working on. (There are probably some people who run when they see me coming!) These clinical stories are about clients who have benefited from music therapy while teaching me and my colleagues how to help others with similar communication challenges.

When music therapists sing with people who have communication difficulties, it is different than a simple "sing-along." In sessions like the ones in this chapter, I am watching the client carefully and making small but important changes to my accompaniment and my singing, such as taking an extra moment after a word so that there is time for the client to set his or her lips and tongue for the next syllable. Sometime I alter my accompaniment to emphasize the beats that aid motor planning and articulation. The non-verbal communication between us is just as important as the words we produce.

September – August
Rochester, New York

"I'm so excited to see what happens," Sandra said, as she and I walked to one of the rooms in our college's speech-language therapy clinic. "I think this is the perfect client to try music therapy."

I had reviewed the client's file. His name was Billy, he was in his 70's, and he loved jazz. He had been coming to the clinic for a couple of years after a stroke left him with no ability to deliberately form words. All that came from his mouth were harshly abbreviated sounds, out of sync with the jerky movements of his lips and tongue. Sandra and some of the other speech-language pathologists (SLPs) on the faculty had been working with him on alternative forms of communication, but Billy -- while friendly and cooperative, -- had not taken to any of these methods consistently.

Billy was already seated at the table in the small treatment room. Across from him was the graduate SLP student assigned to work with him that semester. Sandra took a seat in the corner.

Billy smiled and pointed at my guitar case as I walked in, getting out a strangled "u-h!" as he did. "Yup!" I replied,

"I heard you like music, so we're going to try some today."

I got my guitar out of its case, sat down at Billy's right, and started a blues progression in an R&B style (think B.B. King). The structure had the guitar playing first: a rhythm somewhat like "I'm GO-ing to TEX-as." (bah-DAH dah-dah DUM!) I played four measures of introduction, gradually increasing the volume and energy building up to the vocal entrance.

(bah-DAH dah-dah DUM!)

"I'm sittin' with Billy" I sang using a gritty voice.

(bah-DAH dah-dah DUM!)

"Oh yeeeah!" said Billy, clear as day.

(bah-DAH dah-dah DUM!)

"We're singin' the blues…"

(bah-DAH dah-dah DUM!)

"Yeah, baby!" sang Billy.

(bah-DAH dah-dah DUM!)

"I'm sitting with Billy"

(bah-DAH dah-dah DUM!)

"My, my, yeah!" he added.

(bah-DAH dah-dah DUM!)

"We're singin' the blues"

(bah-DAH dah-dah DUM!)

"Bah –Dah – Beeee!" he sang.

By this point, we were all grinning like fools. I brought the guitar volume down so I could cheer for Billy and consult with my colleagues. Sandra quickly told the graduate student to write down each of the syllables and phonemes that Billy produced as we sang. Off we went into another verse.

***

This was my first chance to work with a client in one of our college clinics. I had taken a job as an assistant professor the previous year but had been focused on finishing my dissertation. Now I had the chance to work in my favorite area: the recovery of speech in people who had survived strokes and traumatic brain injuries. My doctoral work in music therapy and neuroscience had given me many new ideas and it was always a joy to see the effect music therapy had in these circumstances.

Something else that excited me: the chance to work in a place with a minimum of professional territorialism. I've had many great experiences working with speech, physical, occupational and art therapists, and learned so much from their generous and supportive collaboration. However, I've also encountered many people in those professions who are anxious about their own place in the treatment team. Sometimes it is about status and respect. More often it is about money and where the inevitably limited funds will be spent. I understand that. Music therapy makes some of these decisions complicated, because it addresses goals across multiple domains: physical, cognitive, communication, social, emotional, behavioral, spiritual. If a speech therapist is already working on communication goals, the argument goes, why bring in a music therapist to work on the same things? If insurance is only paying for 3 hours of communication work a week, how can the speech therapist give up one of those hours?

My employer, Nazareth College, however, was developing an interprofessional practice that continues today. We have had the chance to do it because our funding is internal, with the clinics in place to train our students and get therapy to underserved people in our community. We aren't beholden to limited insurance funds. We all understand that this isn't currently the reality in hospitals, facilities and home care, but we are committed to educating new generations of therapists and administrators who will see the value for patients and clients of interprofessional work. We have a brand new Wellness & Rehabilitation Institute where physical and occupational therapists, speech-language pathologists, art and music therapists, play therapists, social workers and nurses -- and their students --- can work together.

***

As I brought down the volume for a second time, Billy held his hand up and grabbed a macramé bag he had at his feet. Fishing around inside, he pulled out a slide whistle, kazoo, and harmonica. I looked at Sandra and she laughed. He'd never produced these before, but clearly music was an integral part of his life. I had a harmonica in my bag, so I grabbed it and our next blues round included some back and forth with our instruments. He used all of his and I used my voice to imitate some of the sounds he made. I threw some lyrics to Sandra and the graduate student and they echoed them. It was lively and by the end we were pretty worn out, though happy.

I slowed things down and began a gentle pick pattern on the guitar.

"Michael, row the boat ashore...." I sang, slowing and leaning forward as I started the next word. "Alle....."

"Looooo" sang Billy.

"Ya" I finished. "Michael, row the boat ashore....Alle...."

"Looooo"

"Ya."

It was clear Billy knew and enjoyed the song, so we continued through the traditional verses and did a couple that reflected ourselves. By the final two verses, Billy was singing both of the final syllables himself.

***

Billy had apraxia, a disorder of motor planning. Spoken communication requires both language and speech, with speech being the mechanical production of the words we've chosen and arranged from our language. In almost everyone, the networks for speech and language are based in the left hemisphere of the brain, and when that area is damaged, either speech or language or both can be affected. A disorder of language is called aphasia. People with aphasia can have any of a variety of difficulties, such as finding the words they want or putting all the words of a sentence in the right order. When people who only have aphasia speak, their lips and tongue and breathing work correctly, but the neural network for turning thoughts into words isn't functioning. On the other hand, people who only have apraxia will have a complete coherent thought but they will have damage to the neural networks that coordinate all the motor tasks (breath support, voice, articulation) necessary for speech.

Aphasia and apraxia can, and often do, occur together. Another disorder that can occur after a stroke or brain injury is dysarthria, which manifests as a weakness in the muscles necessary to produce vocal sounds and words. A music therapist can work with clients in all these areas, but it takes a trained speech-language pathologist to assess and distinguish between each disorder. It's then up to the MT-BC to recognize and evaluate what exactly the music is affecting.

The person who first taught me about these distinctions, and about music therapy's role in communication recovery, was Doug.

***

Doug was a patient at the rehabilitation hospital where I worked. He was an extraordinary man: a scientist, an artist, a musician, a loving husband and father. His family was out walking one night when a woman with schizophrenia, off her medication, plowed into them with her car. His young daughter was killed, his young son injured. Doug suffered a severe brain injury.

Doug stayed at our hospital for 9 months, and music therapy was a part of his treatment throughout. When we were playing or listening to music, Doug lit up and you could see and feel the man who had played folk and rock music, the man apart from the injury. Doug was one of the first people I knew who demonstrated the striking difference between the ability to speak and the ability to sing. It was difficult to tell how well Doug understood us, or if he knew what he wanted to say, because he could not coordinate the mechanics of speech. Single syllables were difficult to produce. On the other hand, he could clearly articulate the lyrics of familiar songs. His home town news station came to do a story on his recovery and their video report showed him singing "Slow down...you move too fast....you got to make the morning last -- just kicking down....the cobblestones....lookin' for love and feeling grooooovy!" Each word was pronounced perfectly.

Over the time we worked together, however, I began to realize that perhaps Doug wasn't really processing the meaning of the lyrics. One day, I decided to test this theory. Getting us in a silly mood, with a corny accompaniment on the piano, I had us sing a novelty song, *Yes, We Have No Bananas*. I knew that Doug would know the primary lyrics, as they had been incorporated into a song by one of his favorite singers, Harry Chapin. Sure enough, he began singing immediately, and we sang the main lines over and over again.

Yes, we have no bananas!
We have no bananas today!

After eight repetitions of this chorus, along with some vamping on the word "banana" that Doug picked up on and easily articulated, I stopped. Immediately, I picked up two oversized cards from a large box of photo cards (a common tool used by speech-language therapists).

One of the cards had a photo of a bunch of bananas. The other had a picture of a bath towel.

Without saying anything, I held both photos up, providing some distance between them. I watched Doug look at each photo, shifting his eyes back and forth between them. I hadn't asked him to match the pictures to the lyrics, but knew that anyone who had been singing about bananas for five minutes would naturally gravitate to the corresponding picture.

Doug looked at me quizzically. His expression said, "Why are you showing me these two cards?" He gestured at each and then at me. I could have been holding two pieces of cardboard. Doug could clearly pronounce the words, but the words had no concrete meaning for him. Singing alleviated Doug's apraxia, but it did not significantly help his aphasia. After this experience, I always checked my patients' comprehension of song lyrics, and asked their speech-language therapists to help me assess this. I learned that although many writers use the word "aphasia" as a broad term for communication problems, it was critical for music therapists to understand what we were and were not treating through singing interventions.

***

Billy and I worked together for several semesters at the college clinic, and he helped me develop a way to help a client transition from spontaneous utterances (like his "Oh yeah!") to more intentional speech. The neural networks for well-rehearsed words and phrases (like the alphabet, or a nursery rhyme, or song lyrics) are distinct from the networks used to produce novel, intentional speech (like a food order, or the answer to an interview question). So how could we use the spontaneous success Billy had in music to help him recover some ability to communicate in real world situation? The answer came in a musical format: call and response singing. As Billy voiced words and syllables spontaneously during our music, I would answer him. At first, I imitated him exactly, but then I would take one of his words or syllables (like the "Beee" from his "Bah Dah Bee") and repeat it ("Beee! Beee!"), encouraging him to make the change with me. As he did, he was activating a network in his brain that could produce words or sounds intentionally.

Throughout these exercises, our voices and the guitar or percussion I played intertwined with a musical give and take. The trick in this kind of work is to leave just enough extra room for a response without losing the flow of the music: to sing responses that reflect the client's energy while providing an effective cue. It requires the therapist to be aware of each moment in the musical interaction.

Counselors and psychotherapists know how important it is to be "present" in a session. A therapist must be "in the moment," putting thoughts of the past and future aside. Similarly, the integration of music and musicianship with an effective strategy takes both concentration and flexibility. It's something music therapists learn over time.

***

On another day in the college SLP clinic, Sandra hugged Mavis across the shoulders. "You worked like a trooper today!" Mavis, a petite woman in her 70's, smiled broadly. "And I am going to have to step up my style!" Sandra continued, pointing to Mavis' matching hat and sweater. Mavis was always dressed beautifully when she came to therapy.

"Ok, baby," Mavis said with her usual response, patting Sandra's arm.

"I will figure out a way for us to work on those consonants," I added. "I'll write you a new song to practice."

"Ok, baby," Mavis laughed, and we all smiled as she departed. She was continuing to work diligently on her speech recovery after a stroke three years prior. She was always present for her sessions, even though it was difficult for her to drive and she couldn't always depend on her children for transportation. She used cabs and medical vans when she could, and she almost never missed a session.

My challenge that week was to write a song that would help Mavis work on the final consonants of one-syllable words. Mavis often left them unarticulated after her stroke, making her speech sound slurred and difficult to understand. I wanted to find a way to emphasize those ending sounds without turning them into an additional syllable. I didn't want her saying "ho-puh" for "hope" or "ca-tuh" for "cat."

After work each day, I tried out various meters and styles. Simultaneously, I worked on lyrics; I needed at least 6 practice words per verse. In order to build neural networks to replace or repair damaged ones, the brain must be stimulated repeatedly so the need for a new pathway is intense. Music is a perfect medium for this type of rehabilitation because music makes repetition less tedious -- it can even be fun. Two verses of a song would give Mavis twelve chances to practice the ending consonants, and time would fly in a way that it wouldn't otherwise. In addition, the rhythm of the music would prime the motor networks she needed to form the consonants.

But if Mavis were to make a smooth transition from the music drills to speech outside of her session, the words needed to sound and flow as they would in speech. So I kept working between the music and the lyrics to find a good match. Mavis was not a fan of rock or blues music, so those were out. A waltz (1 – 2 – 3, 1 – 2 – 3) didn't match the lyrics and placed too much emphasis on that last consonant. A two beat measure would let her pronounce the one-syllable word on the first beat with the final consonant landing on the second beat but if those two beats were in a marching style, the final consonant again had an inappropriate emphasis.

As I experimented, I realized that a swing beat would work (think "strawberry" with "straw" drawn out on the first half of the measure and "berry" skipping upwards within the second half). I couldn't know for sure until I tried it with Mavis, though. Every client hears things differently. That's why we work with live music, not with recordings.

I finished up the lyrics; building on something Mavis had told us was one of her regular chores. I would sing the first part of every line, leading up to the downbeat, and Mavis would sing the final word to each line, which would land *on* the downbeat. Each time, she would be learning to include the "p" sound at the end of words. The swing style left pauses of several beats between each line so Mavis wouldn't be overwhelmed.

I need a *mop* (* * * *)
Give me some *soap* (* * * * *)
I won't *stop* (* * * *)
Until the floor is clean

I need a *sip* (* * * *)
of soda *pop* (* * * * *)
I won't *stop* (* * * *)
Until that floor is clean!

As Sandra and I waited for Mavis to arrive at the next session, I played the song and we discussed how to cue the final consonants. I had a student with me, and we decided that she would play a single note on a small glockenspiel on the beat where the "p" sound should be placed. This would provide an auditory cue but not a verbal one, since extra words would get in the way. Between the verses, I would sing a silly chorus so that Mavis could relax between drills.

The door opened and Mavis came in. She was, as usual, dressed in a stylish outfit with a matching hat and scarf, but her mood was noticeably dark. She sat down and we could see that she had tears in her eyes.

"What's wrong, Mavis?" Sharon asked.

Mavis' speech was affected by apraxia, but less so than Billy's. She could get single words and some phrases out. It was harder when she was upset, as she was now.

"No…..no more…can'……dri…." she started. "Daughter….Doc…tor…"

It took a few minutes, but eventually she was able to tell us the story. Her daughter had taken her to the doctor that morning for the conversation children almost inevitably have with their elderly parents: the one where the parent is told they can no longer drive. The daughter had enlisted Mavis' doctor to make this proclamation and Mavis was equally angry with both of them. Her tears were all about the loss of control; being unable to drive and feeling ambushed with that news.

The events of the morning had overwhelmed her and both Sandra and I realized that Mavis would probably not be ready to work. She was continuing to try and tell us details of the doctor's visit as well as the various ways in which this change would be difficult or her. She wanted to talk with sympathetic people more than anything else.

Sometimes it's good just to talk. Though trust is built through music, a music therapy session does not have to be about making music if a conversation will be more therapeutic. On the other hand, creating music that reflects a client's mood and statements can be a wonderfully strong affirmation. Writing a song, for example, can say "what you're telling me is so important that it's worth honoring it." Knowing which direction to go can only happen in the room with the client, and at that moment in the session, I began to strum quietly on my guitar, bringing music into the room without forcing it, and continuing to participate in the conversation.

Mavis noticed. She looked at me curiously and gestured at the guitar. "Wha...?"

I was direct. "Mavis, this is such a difficult day and you're expressing some really strong emotions. I'm wondering how those feelings would sound in a song. I kind of want to sing about it, like this --- "

I demonstrated a minor chord with a determined strum and spoke the words more than singing. "I'm so angry….the doctor told me…." I played a second chord.

"Told me NO!" said Mavis, clearly and smoothly. I quickly reached towards the floor drum I had and struck it three times to echo her words and then returned to my chords.

"I…" and here I hesitated, to show Mavis that I was only suggesting words and she could change them. "I…I don't know how I will get around?"

"Can'…be…" Mavis hesitated, searching for a word (and leaving off the 't' in "can't"). We waited, then Sharon suggested, "independent?" Mavis nodded vigorously.

In this way, we created an eight line verse about Mavis' morning and all the feelings surrounding it. Mavis wrote the chorus herself.

"No one asks me.
They just tell me.
I need my car
To do my things."

We weren't solving the problem, or trying to get Mavis to accept what had happened. We were just honoring her feelings and giving her more ways to get her point across. And when we had sung the song twice and I had played the end with a flourish -- then Mavis was done talking and wanted to work. We actually were able to work on her consonants for half of the session. We knew that she left feeling both heard and accomplished.

***

I first met Letty in the speech-language clinic and worked with her there, but after two years, we started separate sessions in the newly formed music therapy clinic as well. Letty had survived a stroke five years earlier; it had interrupted a strong volunteer career in community service. Letty had mixed aphasia with apraxia, which meant that she had trouble both expressing herself and trouble understanding what others were saying. She could, however, sing familiar melodies in a lovely soprano voice. The lyrics were often garbled, but she usually managed a good approximation of the words that fell at the end of a phrase, on a downbeat.

Her musical ear was remarkable. Letty had taken piano lessons as a child, but had not played as an adult -- and her right arm was not functional after the stroke. Still, when my student and I pulled her up to the electronic piano in her wheelchair one day, she immediately reached out with her left hand and played a C scale. Then, without any cue or help from us, she began to pick out the notes to our usual opening song: *Oh What a Beautiful Morning*. She was not using any kind of muscle memory; she made several mistakes. But slowly and persistently, she picked out the correct notes and soon was able to play the opening melody perfectly.

Persistence was key to Letty's participation in therapy. She wanted to work, to drill on articulation skills like singing "L" words (love, life, laugh). She would make critical sounds as she made errors on the piano, but laugh delightedly when she was successful. And she loved to sing. We often sang just for the joy of it, and we could get giddy, especially singing classic stage songs like *I Could Have Danced All Night*, flinging one arm up in the air at the end like a Broadway diva. She and I developed a rapport that could be described as "the musician and the sane person" -- Letty being the latter. Letty let me know how much she valued my musicianship, and how much she loved laughing at me and anything goofy I did.

After two semesters in music therapy sessions, Letty agreed to come to an additional set of music therapy sessions over the summer to assist me in trying a new approach to integrating music and language recovery. Or, to put it more simply, she agreed to work with me on "yes" and "no."

Many people with mixed aphasia have difficulty using these two words when they want to. If you ask someone like this a question such as, "do you like peas?" or "is your husband's name Bob?" you will often see them give one answer ("no") followed by a shaking of the head as they hear themselves. They will try again, "no....but...yes...wait..." and it will be challenging to discern what their true answer is.

"Yes" and "no" answers are incredibly important if you can't say much else. At the very least, you want to be able to get what you need or want with those two simple words. Letty's comprehension had improved over the years after her stroke (confirmed by the speech-language clinic), so she usually understood simple questions -- but she couldn't consistently convey her opinions and desires when her "yes" and "no" were so inconsistent. How frustrating!

Letty and I were embarking on an experiment to see if we could use music to help not just speech, but language. As I'd seen with Ron and so many other clients, it was possible for a person to sing a familiar song accurately without processing the meaning of the words. If only we all learned songs as children that were functional, that conveyed basic needs. If there were folk songs where the primary lyrics were "I'm thirsty" or rock anthems with a chorus of "I need the bathroom" (that would be something!) then we could likely carry them with us after a brain injury and perhaps use them. Instead, my clients could sing "I could have danced all night" and "Amazing grace, how sweet the sound" and they could enjoy singing, but none of those words helped with fundamental life activities.

So could we use music to help the brain make a connection of meaning with words? The speech-language therapists and faculty said that if I were going to try, I should start with "yes" and "no."

That summer, I developed a protocol that called for Letty to respond to eight basic questions about facts in her life with "yes" responses, and then to respond with "no" to the same questions with incorrect information.

"Is your name Letty?"

"Yes, yes, yes."

and then later:

"Is your name Barbara?"

"No, no, no."

The key was that the music I used for the "yes" questions and answers was significantly different than the music I used for the "no" questions and answers. I hoped to associate a "yes" feeling with one musical idea and a "no" feeling with another. Perhaps, after much repetition, including daily home practice, Letty would, when asked a yes/no question, hear the corresponding music in her head and "sing" the familiar word. Each song had that earworm quality; it was hard to shake after singing it over and over again in the session. Another part of what made the songs memorable was our head nods and shakes and exaggerated formation of the words: "Yes, yes, yes!" or "No, no, no!" Letty laughed when we got especially dramatic.

By the end of our six week summer session, Letty seemed to have gotten the idea and was generating answers consistent with the musical cues. Her aide reported that she was having more success with "yes' and "no" at home. I put my data aside, planning for a formal study with many more participants the next year. (And as so often happens in college life, things got in the way. We are finally starting the study this year.)

That fall, Letty started again in music therapy sessions. As usual, a new semester brought a new student to the sessions. The student would observe and then gradually take over leadership of the sessions. That semester, a graduate student named Pam was assigned to Letty's sessions and because she had several clinical experiences under her belt, I had Pam start leading the opening and closing of Letty's session immediately. Each session was bookended by two songs: we started with *Oh What A Beautiful Morning* and ended with *God Bless America*. Both were songs Letty had been able to sing successfully from the first assessment session, and when I had asked if she would like to sing them in her music therapy sessions, she had told me "yes." Can you guess where this story is going?

Letty's first session was a good start to the semester. She connected with Pam's confident music making and she even tried a new percussion strategy designed to maintain good use of her left arm and hand. As the end of the session approached, I backed off, sitting down at a desk at the side of the clinic and Pam sat down to do the final song, strumming the first chords of the patriotic anthem. I was glancing at some paperwork on the desk when I heard her say, "What's the matter, Letty?" Looking over, I saw Pam stop playing and get Letty's attention. "Don't you want to sing this song?" she queried.

"Try to make your question simpler," I cued Pam.

Pam adjusted. "Letty, do you like singing God Bless America?" she asked.

Letty's head shook dramatically from side to side. "No, no, NO!" she declared.

Uh oh! But also -- wow! It worked! Letty could now tell me what she really thought of the song. I dropped it from our repertoire that week.

CHAPTER NINE

Living and Dying

April - September
Dallas, Texas

The large rectangular great room was already filled with activity when I arrived Saturday morning. The women at this retreat center had arrived the previous evening and would stay until Sunday afternoon. Each had a diagnosis of breast cancer which had metastasized. This weekend, they would have a chance to share their challenges as well as give and receive love and care through journaling, art, movement, and music.

I wasn't there as a therapist, though I'd been asked to participate because of my training and experience. I wouldn't conduct any formal assessments or do any documentation of our time together. I would simply offer what I could to help the women as they requested. That morning, I was available to anyone who wanted to meet as a group and make music.

I checked in with the retreat's leader and one its volunteer coordinators, Deb. They showed me a smaller adjoining room where my group would meet. Comfortable chairs, the ability for everyone to be in a circle, and a door that could give us some privacy. We were all set. By the time the top of the hour arrived, nine women had arrived. It looked like they ranged in age from mid-twenties to late sixties. Many were wearing turbans and scarves, two women were not, two had short curly hair. Several appeared weak, but all were open and friendly, greeting me and each other.

We went around the room and introduced ourselves, and I began by offering a song I had chosen for its ambiguity. It was likely that some of the women present would have strong spiritual beliefs, but also likely that others did not. David Pomeranz's song, *It's In Every One of Us*, lent itself to many interpretations. Even so, after singing the chorus, I told all the participants that if this song wasn't their cup of tea, we'd be sure to find music to their liking before the group was over. I assured them that part of what we could talk about this weekend was how to choose music for different needs, and that those choices were entirely individual. I told them, "There simply isn't any music that affects everyone in the same way, no matter what a clever marketer tries to tell you."

I also shared with the women that I'd long wanted to have some fun making "Music Alert" medical bracelets, like the serious ones that notify people about illnesses or allergies. Mine would list the music I would least want played in my hospital room, in case I was unconscious, and start with the Pachelbel Canon. "Millions of people the world over love that piece of music, but I'd be happy never hearing it again. See what I mean?" I asked them. They certainly did -- and we had a brief silly discussion about both our "guilty pleasures" and least favorite songs. Everyone had a song that was unique to her, and this conversation functioned as a great ice breaker.

I took a couple of moments to share guidelines for the group. I wasn't there to do group therapy, but many of the principles were applicable, including setting some ground rules. No one needs any musical experience to participate, I told them. Music therapy is about the process, not the product. It's okay to cry, and we'd like you to stay, but know you can step out if you need to. We're going to try and stay in the music as much as possible, so see if you can express some things through music as an alternative to talking. I'll be here until noon on Sunday with lots of openings for one-one-one sessions, so don't feel like we have to get everything done right now.

One of the women, Carol, raised her hand. On reflection, she said, she wondered if it would be okay just to come to one of the individual meeting times. She was feeling shaky, both physically and emotionally, and too vulnerable to stay. We all wished her well and I walked her out the door, connecting her with a volunteer.

With everyone else in agreement, I started David's song, teaching them just the chorus and accompanying them on guitar. The song is in 3/4 time – a waltz – and has a gentle flow.

It's in every one of us
To be wise.
Find your heart;
Open up both your eyes.

We can all know everything,
Without ever knowing why.
It's in every one of us,
By and by.

We sang it several times until they were doing it independently. I stood up and took a large hand drum to one of the women who had shown through her body movements that she had a good internal pulse. I was going to show her how to provide a beat under the song, but she took the drum immediately and produced a simple "bah – bah-dah – bah, bah – bah-dah – bah" beat. I gave the woman next to her a long rainstick which produced a whoosh-like background sound as it was turned side to side. Next I picked up several hand chimes and gave one each to six of the women. I had chosen and arranged them so that each pair of women had chimes that, played together, would create a part of the song's harmony. Using hand gestures so as not to interrupt the singing, I had them wait and then play their chimes when I pointed to them.

The women's singing filled the room. I'd chosen a key that they could sing near the range of their speech, so their voices were warm and comfortable. The deep drum gave us a foundation and the rainstick peaceful waves. As each part of the music became second nature, some of the women were able to be almost meditative. After many repetitions, I began signaling them to stop singing, but continue playing their instruments and soon the lyrics faded, but the gentle 3/4 pulse and the rich harmonies of the chimes continued.

I picked up my guitar again and started changing the mood of the music by adding some syncopation. Signaling the chimes to drop out and then the rainstick, the drummer and I continued and as I'd hoped, she was able to pick up the pace just a bit and add a little spice to her rhythms. I didn't know where the music would go, but I wanted the women to hear that we could change direction if we wanted to.

I sang, using just a couple of melody notes, "So we're sitting here…"

Silence from the group, with just the guitar and drum in the space.

Again. "So, we're sitting here…." I looked around, raising my eyebrows and smiling.

"Trying to make music?" offered a woman to my left.

"So we're sitting here…and we're making music…" I sang, looking at my lyricist to see if the change was acceptable. She nodded and smiled. I kept strumming, looking around the room.

"And no one" a voice sang across from me "has thrown up yet!"

Everyone broke into laughter and applauded their peer with the bright purple turban. More members of the group added lyrics and soon we were all singing, chanting, speaking the words as our drummer and I picked up the energy of the accompaniment to match the shared humor.

So we're sitting here
And we're making music
And no one here (no one!)
has thrown up yet!

We might be tired
We might be crazy
But no one here (no one!)
has thrown up yet!

An hour later, the group ended. We had added to the song, and had done some drumming, with everyone playing a rhythm instrument. One of the group had danced for us as we drummed. At the group's request, we finished as we had started, with David Pomeranz's lovely song.

The group headed out to lunch and I straightened up the room. I thought about my oldest friend, Cathy, whom I'd met when I was only three. Cathy had died after fighting a virulent form of breast cancer for a decade, but we had lived so far apart I couldn't be with her near the end. I had to laugh a little, realizing that Cathy would probably have hated a retreat like this. Sharp as a tack and dedicated to her work and family, she had called to sign her sons up for summer swimming lessons the morning of the day she died. But Cathy was not one to be particularly reflective or sentimental -- and the idea of a bonding weekend would have had her running the other way. Everyone faces their challenges differently.

That afternoon and the next morning, I met with several of the women individually. Some wanted to write a song after hearing about the group composition from the previous day. I would not have shared the song myself, because I consider that time confidential (I have altered all the client lyrics in this book), but the group members had been spontaneously singing the song we'd written. Some of the women wanted music recommendations for particular activities: exercise, chemotherapy infusion, getting to sleep. Two of them asked if I could find them a piano teacher, as they'd always wanted to learn to play.

Carol wanted to write a lullaby.

She met with me on Sunday morning. Her son, she told me, was only two years old, and she did not expect to live to see his third birthday. Could we, she asked, write a lullaby and record it, so he could hear her sing to him even after she was gone?

Even as I write this, fifteen years later, I can feel the tears coming. That day, however, Carol was strong and resolute, and I stayed in her space as we wrote the song together. I retrieved my laptop, microphone, and blank CD from my car and sang harmony with her as I accompanied her singing of the lullaby. The art therapist at the retreat helped Carol create a cover for the CD and she left with it that afternoon.

As I packed up to leave for home, Deb -- the volunteer coordinator I had met the previous day -- came to the music room and asked to speak with me. She told me that she loved what Carol had been able to do and wondered if I could help her, as well. She wanted to write a song for her own funeral.

Deb was upbeat and determined. She had some things she wanted to say to her friends and family and just needed help with the musical part of the project. She had a video she wanted me to watch before we composed the song: a news report that had been done about the cancer center where she was being treated. The news crew had filmed a discussion she'd had with her friends and fellow cancer patients about the important things in their lives. Deb had received the raw footage and said we could watch it together before putting down some lyrics. When could I come to her house?

I went the following week. It was summer and I was only working half days at the summer session for my special education students. Deb lived with a roommate in a single story ranch house in a suburb of Dallas. When I arrived, feeling the heat of a Texas summer, she was wrapped up in a blanket on the sofa. "These damn chills," she said. "But screw 'em. Let's get going."

We watched the videotaped discussion and then I got out a notebook. Deb started with the most declarative statements she wanted to include: things like "Pay attention to your life," and "don't let your disagreements fester." When she got stuck, I asked questions and jotted down the words, phrases, and sentences with which she replied. Soon we had three pages of writing, and I pulled out my guitar and portable keyboard. Deb knew that she wanted the song to be lyrical but upbeat, more in a pop style than folk or rock. We experimented with rhythms, major and minor keys, and singing ranges, and I made notes of her preferences.

"So now can you write something for me?" she asked. "I'm getting kind of tired. Can you write something and bring it back to me?"

We agreed that I would do a draft of the song, using the most important messages in the chorus and other thoughts in a verse or two. We set an appointment for the following week.

That is how I found myself sitting on my couch and staring at the notebook of Deb's messages, wishes and hopes. In the present day, I know many music therapists, some of them former students, who work in hospice care and often share the gift of songwriting for goodbyes. At that time, though, I didn't have those connections and I had never been asked to help with something so important. My brain was frozen. I couldn't remember how to write a melody much less an entire song. I stared and prayed.

Suddenly, to my surprise and relief, a melody leapt into my head along with the chords and rhythm that would accompany it. It arrived whole and my only challenge was to find a pen and some staff paper so I could notate it before it disappeared.

The rest of the song flowed after that. At Deb's house the next week, I played it for her and she declared it "Perfect! Done!" That made sense to me. It wasn't my work, it was hers. I'd just been the conduit.

Deb asked me to record the song that day and so I sang it into her portable cassette player and left her with a copy of the music. Her mother told me later that the tape player sat at her bedside as she weakened and she asked to hear the song several times a day up until the afternoon she slipped into a coma.

Five of her friends sang the song with me at Deb's graveside service. We had to laugh when, as we sang to the people gathered for the burial, we were interrupted by church bells from across the street. "Not even in the right key!" one of the friends said afterwards. "That absolutely had to be Deb," said another.

CODA

Annual Conference

November
Louisville, Kentucky

The elevator doors open to the hotel's conference room floor, and I can already hear the slightly muffled sound of drumming coming from down the hall. As I walk along the corridor, my feet begin to match the pace of the beat. I pass a room where the standing-room-only crowd is listening to a presenter and looking at the graphs she has projected on the screen behind her. I hear fragments of her speech -- "decreased anxiety," "four sessions per trial," -- and check the sign on the door: "Application of live vs. recorded music to patients with dementia or Alzheimer's experiencing agitation." I move on. I can hear multiple pitches of drums now, and a driving, syncopated rhythm. I'm outside the door now and as the volume increases, the playing becomes more frenzied until...WHAM! A final loud beat and then cheering from the participants. Several of us in the hallway smile at each other, remembering the time when we last took part in a session like that.

Now that the drumming has stopped, I can hear various sounds coming from the exhibit hall around the corner. Chords from a piano. Strums from a harp. Chimes. I'm anxious to get a chance to wander the hall, checking out the newest books, instruments and electronics, but I have meetings all afternoon, so it will have to wait until this evening.

It's the second day of the American Music Therapy Association's annual conference -- or rather, the second day of regular presentations. Many of us have been here for two pre-conference days of meetings and are continuing to meet in committees, boards, and the Assembly, with our fellow voting delegates from around the country. Music therapists are not nearly as numerous as speech-language pathologists or physical therapists (there are about 7,000 board-certified music therapists in the U.S.) but our profession is organized and run in a similar way. Our therapists adhere to documents like a Code of Ethics and Scope of Practice. Our college and university programs must have the curriculum and resources to help students achieve "professional competencies" and become board-certified. Therapists in advanced training must demonstrate specific higher-level skills in research or clinical techniques.

***

For many years, as a new and then slightly more experienced therapist, I attended the annual conference primarily to attend presentations. Some presenters described research that I could apply to my clients; some taught me how to do particular interventions. There were also speeches on music therapy theory that helped me understand and develop my own approach. After a few years, I joined a committee, but still, the majority of my time was spent learning. During those first years, I would sometimes almost dread attending a session presented by a therapist working with clients similar to mine. I would approach the session assuming I would discover how backward and archaic my approach was. Of course, like most of my colleagues, I usually discovered that I was on the right track after all, and I could relax and pick up some new ideas.

There are always some sessions in which potentially valuable information is buried in a poor presentation: slides with indecipherable type, a speaker with a droning voice, or a speaker whose text is obscured by "um" and "you know" and more recently, So..." Other sessions have titles that have nothing to do with the content. And there is the inevitable dilemma of choosing what to attend when there is more than one interesting session scheduled at the same time. This kind of thing happens in any profession's conferences.

What makes a music therapy conference different, I've found, is its energy -- and that naturally comes from having music all around us. Even more than other music conferences, the electricity at a music therapy conference comes from the spontaneity and creativity in the production of the music. Musical expression pops up everywhere, from singing in the line for registration to a capella harmony by folks waiting for a presentation, to the evening cabarets and drum circles. Furthermore, the relative small size of our profession means that after a few years, it feels like we really do all know each other. It's impossible to walk down a hallway in the conference area and not hear someone cry out "Oh my gosh!! You're here!!" or "Yay! The band is back together!"

I present at our annual conference every year, sometimes with colleagues, sometimes on my own. I am a problematic partner for a presentation (or writing project) because I tend to mull things over for weeks or months, scribbling notes on napkins or the borders of departmental meeting agendas, only writing the final text and preparing slides the week or the day before the presentation. Poor Kathleen dealt with this all the years of our SEMTAP presentations and now it's often my fellow professors who find themselves coping with this selfish work style.

The presentations usually go well, however, because I'm just crazy about what I do for a living, and I gained a lot of experience in communicating that during my travels with the publishing company. I wander from side to side as I talk, if the session allows it, and I gesture enough that any fellow speaker probably has to bob and weave to get out of the way. I talk fast, but clearly. It works, most of the time.

***

Washington DC, 1999: the 9th World Congress of Music Therapy. I had been invited to present on the SEMTAP at a day-long institute on assessment. I was fourth on a program of four presenters, and the other three were distinguished experts from music therapy, medical administration, and certification agencies. By the time my slot arrived, the audience had spent a morning and afternoon awash in data and statistics: important and helpful information, all of it, but a lot to take in. The end of the institute and the promise of a full meal were on everyone's mind. I was still wondering how I had ended up on the program and wondered what the audience would think of my more prosaic, pragmatic content after such detailed and serious presentations. At least, I thought, my presentation is lively!

I dove into my subject matter, using my usual style. I saw some grateful looks from audience members who adjusted themselves in their seats, waking up a bit. One participant sitting next to the center aisle, however, had a different reaction. After I'd been speaking for a few minutes, I saw his arm stretch out into the aisle and his hand, flat and parallel to the floor, pump slowly up and down -- a virtual brake pedal. Still worried that my listeners would drift off from fatigue or hunger or both, I kept up my pace. What I didn't notice was the translator for a group of Spanish-speaking attendees to my right. After the first 20 minutes, however, I paused to look down at my notes -- and before I could get going again, I saw the translator waving at me.

"Could you stop for just a minute, please? I need to catch up."

She turned to her group and proceeded to talk for what seemed like 5 minutes, though I'm sure it was shorter than that. However long it lasted, it became funny for all of us, including those getting the translation. It was clear something had to give. I decided I had to keep going, so I quickly promised a transcript to those who wanted one, and offered to stay afterwards for questions. That settled, I was off to the races once more.

At the end of the presentation, the owner of the stretched-out hand came up to me, and I recognized him as a professor from one of the colleges in the southeast. In a slow, leisurely drawl, he said, "Now, I know why you thought you needed to go so fast, but I just wanted to let you know ... some of us can't think as fast as you talk."

He smiled mischievously and walked away.

***

"Betsey! Yay!" I hear from one of the tables along the side of the wide corridor. It's a dear friend from my Texas years and our hug is the best part of the day so far. We sit and chat, soon joined by a couple of other Texas music therapists. Facebook and other social media have helped us keep in touch more than we used to be able to, but there's still no substitute for seeing each other.

Today we find ourselves reminiscing about the conference in California in November of 2001; more lightly attended after 9/11, but even more memorable as we supported each other with music.. We were so proud of our association's disaster relief team, which provided many services to first responders, grieving families and others affected by the tragedy. We laugh, too, however, as we remember an exhibitor that year who was demonstrating a supposedly miraculous technique using autoharps, claiming that by placing the autoharp on a person's chest and strumming it while chanting, she could repair the muscle tone of a child with cerebral palsy, help a learning disabled student coordinate the hemispheres of his brain, and improve the sight of someone with a visual impairment. We still recall the cacophony of that exhibit booth, as autoharps tuned to different keys were demonstrated simultaneously by the exhibitors. They were *not* invited to return the following year.

We share notes on upcoming sessions and I beg for proxies at a couple of presentations I wish I could attend. This year, like many of the therapists that have been around as long as I have, I am spending much of the conference at meetings. I am the co-chair of our Ethics Board and I sit on the Academic Program Approval Committee. I'm participating in a task force that is reviewing advanced competencies, and as an alternate to the Assembly, I've been called up due to an absence.

One might think this would be a dreary conference for me, but the truth is, our profession comes alive for me in these meetings -- differently than in practice, to be sure, but powerfully in its own way. Every advance of the profession through research and practice must be conveyed to our upcoming students, so reviewing our academic programs is critical. The complications that social media can bring to confidentiality and therapeutic relationships must be addressed in the Code of Ethics. This year, the Assembly is discussing the idea that we should move our certification requirements from a bachelor's degree to a master's degree because of the increasing breadth of knowledge and musical skills necessary for effective practice. I'm one of many in favor of this change, but there are colleagues I respect who disagree.

A student of mine from Nazareth stops by and I get her to sit down and meet everyone. Alison is a junior and she is already participating in leadership through the national student association. She is a talented oboist and has just finished a clinical placement where I supervised her work with a girl who survived a traumatic brain injury. She eventually wants to work with at-risk teens. My own experience has taught me that networking is crucial in a profession as small as ours. I want my colleagues to know how special this student is, in case she wants to apply for an internship or future job in their area.

All around us at other tables, ideas are being shared and connections formed, so much so that the breaks between sessions and meetings sometimes offer even more information and possibilities than the presentations themselves. And always, somewhere nearby or in the distance, there is music making. My therapist friends and I, hearing a familiar melody from a presentation in a closed room across the hall, begin harmonizing with it and laughing as we secretly contribute to the song. We encourage my student to join us, beginning what we hope will be a long association as colleagues and friends.

ACKNOWLEDGEMENTS

How can I possibly thank all the people who have helped me find this career and flourish in it? Inevitably this will be an incomplete list. My thanks go to all of these people and many more.

- To my family, who made me musical and curious – the perfect combination.
- To my clients and their families, who have taught me all the most important things about music therapy.
- To my colleagues from Texas: Baylor, Birdville and beyond, who have been my teachers, mentors and friends, always encouraging and inspiring.
- To my teachers, who encouraged my curiosity and kept me on a forward path.
- To my students past and present, who have asked so many interesting questions and are making such a difference in the world.
- To my friends outside of music therapy, who make me laugh and make sure I'm more than my work. Many thanks to those of you who read drafts and gave helpful feedback -- and hugs to Karen, who took care of all the things I was neglecting while I hunched over my computer.

- To Kathleen Coleman, who first taught me, then supported me, then created with me, always with infinite patience. We've done some good things, my friend!
- To Milton Goldberg and Dorothy DeLay, who were my teachers at the beginning and end of my violin career. You are gone now, but your words are always in my music.
- To Sandy, Charlie, Wayne, and Kelly: though you may not know it, each of you helped me live a different dream.
- To the jazz trio, Phronesis, whose CDs *Alive* and *Life to Everything* were the perfect background to my writing sessions.
- To everyone at Nazareth College where I finally found a place that fits. I'm grateful for the interprofessional and interdisciplinary collaboration and the time and support to write this book.
- And looking back on the last six years in particular, I'm especially thankful for Laurie Keough: the perfect colleague and a blessing every day.

READING AND LINKS

To learn more about the music therapy profession, how to become a music therapist, upcoming conferences, recent news and more:

> The American Music Therapy Association
> www.musictherapy.org

To learn about board-certification and the music therapy Scope of Practice:

> The Certification Board for Music Therapists
> www.cbmt.org

For international music therapy information:

> The World Federation of Music Therapy
> http://www.musictherapyworld.net/

Peer-reviewed journals (a selection):

> Journal of Music Therapy
> http://jmt.oxfordjournals.org/

> Music Therapy Perspectives
> http://mtp.oxfordjournals.org/

Nordic Journal of Music Therapy
British Journal of Music Therapy
Australian Journal of Music Therapy

The following publishers specialize in academic books about music therapy:

Barcelona Publishers
https://www.barcelonapublishers.com

Jessica Kingsley
www.jkp.com

The American Music Therapy Association
http://www.musictherapy.org/bookstore/

Prelude Music Therapy: home of the SEMTAP and other materials for music therapists and people working with children with special needs
www.preludemusictherapy.com

Nazareth College (including the Music Therapy program and the Wellness & Rehabilitation Institute)
www.naz.edu

CPSIA information can be obtained
at www.ICGtesting.com
Printed in the USA
FFOW04n1512280816
27113FF